Mental Health in Remote Rural Developing Areas

Concepts and Cases

Mental Health in Remote Rural Developing Areas

Concepts and Cases

Formulated by the
Committee on Therapeutic Care

Group for the Advancement of Psychiatry

Report No. 139

Published by

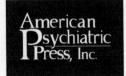

American Psychiatric Press, Inc.

Washington, DC
London, England

Published by American Psychiatric Press, Inc.
1400 K Street, N.W., Washington, DC   20005

Library of Congress Cataloging-in-Publication Data
Group for the Advancement of Psychiatry. Committee on Therapeutic
  Care.
  Mental health in remote rural developing areas : concepts and
cases / formulated by the Committee on Therapeutic Care, Group for
the Advancement of Psychiatry.
      p.   cm. — (Report ; no. 139)
    ISBN 0-87318-207-3 (alk. paper)
    1. Rural mental health services.   2. Rural mental health services—
Case studies.   3. Rural mental health services—Alaska—Case
studies.   4. Rural mental health services—Developing countries—
Case studies.   I. Title.   II. Series: Report (Group for the
Advancement of Psychiatry : 1984) ; no. 139.
    [DNLM: 1. Community Psychiatry—Alaska.   2. Community
Mental Health Services—Alaska.   3. Rural Health—Alaska.   W 1 RE209BR
no. 139 1995 / WM 30.6.G8823m 1995]
RC321.G7 no. 139
[RC451.4.R87]
616.89 s—dc20
[362.2'0425]
DNLM/DLC
for Library of Congress   95-33219
                                                                               CIP

British Library Cataloguing in Publication Data
A CIP record is available from the British Library.

Contents

Preface

Seventy-five percent of the world's population lives in "developing countries" or in rural locations that lack most standard mental health services. Many of these areas are beginning to be industrialized, modernized, and urbanized and are gaining access to specialized high-technology health care. The transitions associated with increasing development, however, often bring in their wake social pathology and behavioral lifestyle problems; these include breakdowns in traditional social norms and community supports, family violence, alcoholism, cultural identity problems, and perceived inability to control one's environment and daily life.

Biomedical technology alone, despite its dramatic accomplishments in solving some health problems, has not been as successful in dealing with the social and behavioral problems that come with economic development and the opening up of formerly isolated cultures. New approaches are needed, involving social sciences as well as medical disciplines, multidisease perspectives, multiple levels of analysis, more sensitive development strategies, and more collaboration between urban specialists and people in rural developing areas. Family, community, and environmental concerns need to be better integrated with psychiatric and biomedical techniques. Additional attention to the social, behavioral, and cultural determinants of change in health-related issues is required.

In this book, representative types of problems in remote rural communities in Alaska are presented, with discussion of principles and attempted solutions. Like many Third World locations, these Alaskan communities have been treated as "territories" by people outside the region who are primarily interested in rapid development of such natural resources as gold, timber, and oil. The "bush villages" still have to cope with inadequate transportation and communication infrastructure, housing and sanitation problems, low educational levels, poverty, high rates of certain infectious diseases, and lack of professional human resources. Access to even basic health care is limited; most services are provided by paraprofessionals in village clinics, with sicker patients having to be flown out to distant rural towns for treatment.

Alaskan villagers are also coping with the social fallout from cultural changes that have taken place. As in other developing areas, there are high rates of social and behavioral health problems such as alcoholism, child abuse, suicidal behavior, and domestic violence.

Weather and lack of transportation make it difficult for psychiatrists in "bush" Alaska to see their patients. Once physical access to services is achieved, the problems are just beginning. Another kind of "remoteness" is created by language barriers and by differences in culture, values, and lifestyle. There are community-wide as well as individual problems. Local people may feel loss of control; political, legal, and economic disenfranchisement; disruption of traditional lifestyles; and inability to control their environment.

Because resources are limited, and standard approaches often do not work, the utmost creativity and flexibility are required to develop new types of programs.

In this book, we illustrate some of the social and environmental influences that shape health and mental health care, using examples from rural villages in Alaska as well as other developing areas of the world. The focus is on problems that are of special interest to psychiatrists. Because most developing areas face extremely basic problems such as malnutrition, lack of adequate sanitation, and high rates of infectious diseases, relatively little attention has been paid to the mental health aspects of their situation. Alaska provides some unique opportunities; its isolated villages have many of the same problems found in the Third World, but its greater resources allow some attempts to provide mental health services.

The cases and discussions focus on the role of the public psychiatrist, who, in these settings, often has limited ability to pick and choose which problems to deal with and who also has multiple options for conceptualizing a problem and taking action. The cases illustrate such topics as how to develop aftercare and follow-up plans for chronic mentally ill patients who live in remote areas, how to help remote rural general hospitals manage psychiatric patients better, what to do when totally new service systems need to be developed, and how to deal with interprofessional conflicts that can arise when staffing is very limited. Methods of working with paraprofessionals, who often provide much of the primary care in remote locations, are discussed, as well as family problems, cultural issues, and problems in the patient's wider environment that can affect treatment. Issues of epidemiology, how to use a variety of social science methods, how to respond when psychiatric conditions seem influenced by legal and environmental changes, ways to analyze the kinds of problems that are encountered, and comments on consultation methods and training and supervision issues are also included.

Psychiatrists in remote rural areas may be called on to function as clinicians, assessing difficult clinical situations and advising on complicated treatment plans. The psychiatrist may play other, additional roles, however, functioning at various times as systems builder, program developer, specialized backup for local response teams and service networks, coach and trainer, quality assurance expert, and researcher.

Approaches described in the book include extensive use of community education, to encourage local people to maintain healthy lifestyles; self-help techniques; use of paraprofessional emergency response teams; team efforts with local primary care physicians; use of local advisory boards to help set resource allocation priorities and coordinate care; development of local teams to work on specific problems such as fetal alcohol syndrome; development of "mental health dictionaries" to ease translation problems; development of "Spirit Programs" to help strengthen traditional cultural values; and consultation by telephone. These methods all build on local capacity, with the goal of getting the maximum services possible for the limited money and psychiatric professional time that are available.

People who have not spent much time studying the issues in rural mental health care often seem to assume that the main rural problem is lack of access to the technology and specialists available in urban centers; they see the main challenge as how to transfer or export urban know-how to less developed locations.

Some "rural" locations have considerably more resources and are less isolated than the Alaskan village settings. For such areas, exporting technology and specialists from urban centers is often feasible, and such approaches are described in the community mental health literature (Cutler and Madore 1980; Libo and Griffith 1968). In this book, the terms *remote rural* and *developing areas* are used to indicate settings where the problems are not just those of access and lack of resources, but are of a qualitatively different nature.

Rural mental health is seen by many as a low-status, peripheral field, and it tends to get relatively little attention within mainstream psychiatry. Something on the periphery can, of course, be "marginal" or "leading edge," depending on how one looks at it.

The rural mental health literature sometimes contributes to the field's low status and peripheral position, reciting a list of "ain't it awful" frustrations and failing to challenge the usefulness of current urban models. Descriptions tend to stay within one country's boundaries, so that cultural, political, and economic aspects of problems are not apparent. Because a broad, interdisciplinary focus is rarely employed, rural mental health remains something that only happens out "in the boonies."

Yet a consideration of mental health in remote rural locations raises important questions about underlying premises and assumptions of current psychiatric practice—diagnostic issues in different cultural groups, how certain types of problems should be conceptualized, who or what should be treated, and basic values and world views.

There are a lot of people out there with similar problems, in locations within developed nations such as the United States and Western European countries as well as the developing areas (Appleby and Araya 1991; Giel and Harding 1976; Green 1991). As population mobility increases around the globe, the kinds of problems described in Alaska acquire greater relevance to all of us. In the United States, for example, the population of foreign-born immigrants and refugees is escalating rapidly and changing in composition. An estimated 1.2 million immigrants, both legal and illegal, arrived in 1993 alone, 80% of whom are people of color. Many are poor and poorly educated, with fewer than 50% having a high school education.

At the same time, many people dislocated from remote rural settings within the United States are migrating into the cities. Even psychiatrists who work in metropolitan settings are likely to encounter "urban villagers" who retain the values and understandings of their home communities.

Multinational economic projects have already fostered more contacts and relationships between developed and developing countries. Health problems too, such as acquired immunodeficiency syndrome (AIDS), drug abuse, and some pollution problems, are "transnational" in scope. Better understanding of social and behavioral dimensions in developing countries will be essential for effective solutions.

This book should therefore be of interest not only to psychiatrists but to many others, in a number of disciplines and in different countries and work settings. Its purpose is to stimulate awareness and discussion of a "frontier" still waiting to be adequately scouted and explored.

Dedication

At the time of publication, the Group for the Advancement of Psychiatry was informed of the untimely death of Dr. William W. Richards, whose leadership and dedication brought this manuscript to completion. The Committee on Therapeutic Care dedicates this book to his memory.

Acknowledgments

We acknowledge the many individuals who provided valuable assistance to members of the Therapeutic Care Committee of the Group for the Advancement of Psychiatry. These include many state, federal, and tribal organizational staff at multiple facilities throughout Alaska, who participated in interviews, shared their experiences, and tried to teach us about "remote rural mental health." The views expressed here represent those of the members of the Therapeutic Care Committee and do not reflect official positions of state, federal, or tribal organizations.

Special thanks to Maribeth Richards for patiently typing up multiple drafts of the text and to Carol Barkin for expert editing of our text. We also acknowledge many institutions—including Bethesda Oak Hospital; Pennsylvania Hospital; and the universities of North Carolina, West Virginia, and Pittsburgh—which supported the participation of members in this consultation activity.

Introduction

The term *health transition*, coined by John Caldwell, describes the changes that occur as formerly remote and isolated areas have increasing contact with the outside world and go through a development process (Chen et al. 1992); it encompasses those changes in social norms, social structure, and individual behavior that result in better health (Caldwell et al. 1990). The following three scenes provide an illustration of the concept of "health transition."

Examples of "Health Transition"

Scene One

A doctor in a developing country in Africa is responsible for 76,000 people. He sees 1,000 patients and delivers 85 babies per month, handling malaria cases, burns, broken bones and cuts from accidents, gunshot wounds, kidney problems, and premature twins. The hospital he works in lacks air-conditioning, incubators for premature births, and oxygen for resuscitation. There is no safe blood supply. The doctor also lacks access to medical journals, and continuing medical education is rarely available to him.

There is little time to address his patients' more specialized needs, such as psychiatric conditions or the many family problems he sees. The villagers speak an African dialect, and describing their psychiatric conditions in the standard nomenclature poses major translation problems.

About 30 cents per capita per year is spent on health in this country, and the average person makes somewhere between 0.1 to 0.3 visits per year for a health check at the clinic. The rest of the time he or she may try various self-help approaches, visit a local folk healer, or just go untreated until the problems become extremely severe. Rates of infant mortality and many infectious diseases are very high; life expectancy is in the low 50s.

The local people see many of their health problems as created by neocolonialists; they believe these outsiders want to exploit their country's natural resources without paying the costs of responsible and ecologically sound development. They perceive land reform issues and other political and economic problems as very much connected with their health problems and lack of health services.

Scene Two

A small 16-bed general hospital, with 6 family physicians, 13 nurses, and a budget of $4,000,000, covers a rural region in Alaska. Staff are in public service on government salaries. The hospital serves 7,000 people, scattered in remote villages up to an hour or so away by airplane, with no road access. The villages, of 100–600 people, have small health clinics staffed by paraprofessionals. These village workers, known as village health aides or community health practitioners, do many of the jobs that the doctor described in Scene One does. They have minimal training, but can phone the regional family physicians at the hospital for backup. Difficult cases are flown in to the hospital. A psychiatrist visits the region every 3 months for a specialty clinic. Social workers and a psychiatric nurse stationed in the same town as the hospital provide some itinerant services to the villages.

Nobody is quite sure what the overall cost of the health services is, because there is a confusing mix of federal, state, and local programs, with various categorical budgets and overlapping responsibilities. It might well be $2,000 per person per year or more, if all the costs were figured in, with an average of about four to six visits per person per year to the health system.

As in Scene One, there are still many health problems from infectious diseases. The tuberculosis epidemic of the 1940s and 1950s in

Alaska has been vanquished, but problems like hepatitis B are a major concern. Life expectancy is in the high 60s to low 70s—better than that in Scene One, but still lower than many places. The mortality of newborns is low, because of good obstetric care, but once the women leave the hospital with their babies, many of them have problems at home, and postnatal mortality is high. In addition to the kinds of health problems described in Scene One, there are increasing numbers of people with chronic illness, which often seems related to lifestyle patterns. There are rising lung cancer rates because people still smoke a lot, many alcohol-related problems, high rates of family violence, and rising rates of adult-onset diabetes associated with changes from the traditional diet and exercise. There are also high rates of sexually transmitted diseases, teen pregnancies, and suicide.

Many other psychiatric and family problems are common in the villages, and staff have minimal resources to deal with them. Very serious psychiatric cases are sent out on expensive plane rides to psychiatric hospitals in distant cities, but soon come back home with their problems not much changed. Most of the villagers speak some English, but the older people speak mainly their own native languages and appear to have very different concepts of mental disorder than most psychiatrists have.

The villagers have strong feelings about the outside developers who have come into the state, creating major changes in every aspect of their lifestyle while extracting natural resources like gold and oil for export. In the health field, efforts are being made to gain local control of the health system that has been operated in the past by the government, with the goals of self-determination and health programming that fits the local priorities better and is more culturally sensitive.

Scene Three

A big-city program in the United States has the kinds of medical and psychiatric services that most of us are used to. Various options for service are available, some of which are "managed care" and limit psychiatric visits to a certain number per year. The costs run $3,800 or more per patient per year. Psychiatrists are available at a ratio of one for every 8,000 people; teaching hospitals and universities are nearby. Concerns about malpractice litigation, as well as licensing and credentialing problems, limit what paraprofessionals can do. People have longer life expectancies than earlier generations, and infant mortality and infectious disease rates are lower. Heart disease, cancers, and problems associated with chronic disease have increased, because people are living longer, and there are high rates of lifestyle-related problems such as drug abuse and violence. In many pockets of the community, access to care seems to be low or almost nonexistent. Language and translation problems are still present for certain subgroups, but for many everything can be done in English.

In this city as in other areas of the country, considerable debate has arisen over who should be responsible for, and how best to approach, problems that involve social factors (e.g., housing, education, job opportunities) or lifestyle aspects (e.g., substance abuse, sexually transmitted disorders). The general public sees some of these as related to health or mental health, but doctors are wary of medicalizing social pathology and promising more than they can deliver in the way of interventions.

Health Transition

Although health transition is associated with changes in epidemiological patterns and in mortality, the focus is on the social processes through which a society improves its health and life expectancy. Consistent with the emphasis on the social determinants of health, the concept of health transition defines health as more than the absence of disease; it is construed as the ability to function. Dubos' (1965) definition of health as a "physical and mental state fairly free of discomfort and pain which permits persons to function effectively and as long as possible in the environment" works well in this context.

The social dimensions most relevant to health transition are the perception of and the ability to control one's environment and daily life so that health is maintained. Societies in the early stages of health transition tend to enforce long-standing social controls that prescribe certain behaviors for dealing with illness and maintaining health. As the transition progresses, social and community structures change to incorporate additional health-seeking and health-maintenance behaviors. This social transformation is the key to the health transition process (Findley 1992).

Strategies used by modernized, technologically superior groups to develop local resources can easily alter traditional social controls. This is the story frequently replayed in colonies, on plantations, in territories, and in the modern equivalents—developing countries with low labor costs and/or natural resources that more developed countries want to export.

Problems such as those in rural Alaska described in this book are really in a middle zone—between those faced by developing countries in the Third World and those familiar to many psychiatrists who work in large "First World" metropolitan areas.

Three Stages of Health Transition

The first stage of health transition is characterized by high levels of infectious and parasitic diseases. In the context of malnutrition and generally poor health, children experience high mortality risks, life expectancy is short, and high mortality and high morbidity coexist. The total disease burden is high.

In the second stage of health transition, the major infectious epidemics are substantially reduced. Mortality begins to fall, but morbidity may not yet decline proportionately. In today's transitional countries, although water- and airborne infectious diseases are decreasing, parasitic diseases (e.g., malaria, leprosy, leishmaniasis, filariasis, onchocerciasis, schistosomiasis) are still prevalent.

In the third stage of the transition, water- and airborne infectious diseases and parasitic diseases have a much lower incidence. They are replaced, however, by higher rates of chronic, degenerative, or accident-related diseases. Because many of these diseases have low incidence rates among young children, the childhood years tend to be more disease-free. Levels of illness in the population rise with age, however, due to accidents and to diseases related to the human-made environment or to aging. For example, there are high rates of cardiovascular disease and malignant neoplasms. This is the stage when psychiatrists and other mental health professionals are apt to be called on to do something about high rates of alcoholism, suicides, violence, and other behavioral lifestyle-related problems that are defined as "mental health" problems.

During the transition, socioeconomic inequalities and regional developmental differences may result in marked heterogeneity in the tempo of health change. At any given time, some groups will be experiencing the disease and mortality patterns of the earlier stages, while others will be subject to the later transitional diseases. Some populations may exhibit signs of multiple stages simultaneously: in Sao Paulo, Brazil; Bombay, India; and many Alaskan villages, residents bear the burdens of both poverty and industrial pollution, and they may experience acute respiratory infections as well as degenerative diseases and numerous chronic behavioral health problems.

Another factor is the transition from diseases caused by natural infection processes to those that are largely consequences of the human-made environment. In an early transitional stage, the population faces significant mortality risks early in life. In later stages, the significant health problems emerge later, when the cumulative effects of aging or exposure to various pollutants manifest themselves. In the intermediate stages, childhood morbidity due to acute infectious diseases is usually lower, but childhood and adult morbidity related to parasitic or recurrent infectious diseases is likely to be high.

In the initial stage, educational and public health measures are directed at infectious and communicable diseases that can be reduced by prudent measures to ensure a safe source of water, appropriate management of waste products, adequate sanitation, and preventive health care. Since these approaches are both focused and effective, impressive advances can occur relatively quickly, with sharp reductions in infant, child, and maternal mortality.

Scene One is at an early stage of the health transition process, with low life expectancies; much infectious disease; high infant mortality; and other problems such as lack of food, poor sanitation and housing, and low literacy rates. In such situations, environmental changes (e.g., improvements in food supplies, better sanitation, safe water) can often make more difference to health statistics than high technology, hospital-based, specialized care.

Scene Two, set in rural Alaska, might look quite backward if compared with urban programs with high technology and specialized care. Compared with Scene One, however, it is very rich indeed. It has many of the problems of developing areas; the villagers still have to contend with inadequate housing, poor sanitation, limited school systems, political inequities, lack of jobs, and various cultural issues. In this book, such a situation is called "remote rural" because most of the literature on "rural" mental health deals with areas far less isolated than those in Alaska. Remoteness may also stem from social class, cultural and language differences, and feelings about enforced dependency on outsiders.

The villages in Scene Two have more resources, and more access to specialty backup, than the situation portrayed in Scene One. Professionals in Scene Two are contending with issues that are familiar in some other rural contexts, but are "out of sight, out of mind" in big-city practices. In terms of health transition, these villages have partially completed the process, still retaining a lower life expectancy and high rates of certain infectious diseases and some forms of infant mortality, but also showing more of the "diseases of civilization" that seem to be considerably influenced by social factors and lifestyle patterns. Patients may get a fair amount of information about their physical conditions from family physicians in this type of general hospital setting, but less obvious cognitive factors may not be explored or explained. Thus, despite some years of contact with modern health systems, there can still be surprising differences between what the patient believes and what doctors assume when it comes to psychiatric disorders.

In Scene Three, in terms of health transition, the bulk of the population is now living longer and getting more chronic diseases. Problems stemming from environmental factors such as lack of food and poor sanitation are decreasing, and most infectious diseases are under better control. Resources are more available, although distribution of and access to these resources are skewed. Psychiatric services can be much more highly specialized at this stage of the health transition process.

Common processes seem to be at work in all three scenes. Social and environmental problems are interacting with health concerns, and the medical system is limited in what it can do. Psychiatric problems, and especially the preventive and early intervention aspects, tend to get relatively little attention even in the most richly funded metropolitan centers.

Implementation of Health Transition

Implementation of the first stage of health transition usually requires some degree of community mobilization through a set of attitudes that might be called "psychological modernity," as well as the rudimentary organization of primary health care (Mechanic 1992). Some degree of modernity is needed to motivate the population to use primary health care facilities, to cooperate in care, and to follow advice and instruction. However, the necessary level of modernity and the educational experience it depends on is relatively modest if the system of primary care is economically, physically, and culturally accessible and if it maintains a preventive orientation with aggressive community outreach. A well-organized system of care can have impressive results even in highly traditional contexts.

The later stages of health transition encompass a broader segment of the life cycle, a multiplicity of diseases with varying causes, and less proven social and technological interventions. They pose more difficult challenges. Progress in these stages is likely to depend to a greater extent on the degree of psychological modernity and the quality of social organization. Diet, work and environmental risks, accidents, and high-risk behaviors are some of the issues that must be dealt with.

Within each society some people adapt more quickly to changes and could be said to "modernize" faster. These people adopt different social roles: they tend to be more active in politics, practice birth control more regularly, have fewer children, adopt innovative practices sooner, appear more productive by the standards of the outsiders, keep their children in school longer and encourage them to take up more technical occupations, and press more actively for social change. This group is of great interest to anyone doing community development work, because its members can be extremely helpful in taking on social transformation roles if convinced of the value of a new development.

The single most important factor associated with psychological modernity is formal schooling. Its importance may derive not from curricula but from responding to ordered sequences of activities and scheduling, modeling and other psychosocial processes in the classroom, cognitive complexity, sense of mastery, aggressiveness in seeking information, conceptual skills in managing information, and learning to cope more actively with complex situations.

Only a small amount of health-relevant behavior seems to be governed by conscious motives. Much of the behavior is shaped by norms and routine activities that may inadvertently contribute to or damage health. Health is a derivative of the everyday structure of routines, activities, and socioeconomic circumstances.

Thus, promoting health in the later stages of health transition is much more difficult than in the early stages, because it is an exercise in changing culture. The challenge is to introduce modern attitudes with minimal disruption of the web of relationships, loyalties, and dependencies that exists in a given cultural setting. Rapid modernization and technical change often result in generational conflict, disruption of traditional culture, and high levels of anomie and alienation. These effects contribute to personal pathology and violence. The traditional web of helping relationships and patterns of sustenance should not be torn apart during attempts at modernization. Health-enhancing environments must deal not only with the issues of economic subsistence but with the broader context of cultural integrity, group structure, and personal meanings.

Over the long term, the issue then is how to encourage the evolution of psychological modernity in a way that minimizes cultural dislocations and personal anomie.

The term *mental health* carries an expanded meaning in the context of health transition. It is broader than standard clinical psychiatry and broader even than *community mental health*. The important difference is that total systems-based interventions are needed, rather than clinical interventions or approaches limited to "basic services" provided by the typical community mental health center or social agency. Different models of care, the filling of new roles, and a reorientation of the mental health professional's thinking are required.

Health and Mental Health Enhancement

The cases in this book illustrate a range of social and behavioral health problems found in transitional settings. This is why situations that at first might not seem "psychiatric"—dealing with social and cultural norms in villages, family and institutional problems, legal and religious issues—are included along with individual case studies.

To affect health in these locations significantly, cooperation is needed among various disciplines, and multiple levels of analysis and multidimensional approaches to problems are useful. Figure 1–1 illustrates a health and mental health enhancement model, with different levels of analysis (adapted from Weiss 1992):

1. Intrapersonal level. At the intrapersonal level, the focus is on the individual (e.g., genetic background, constitution, developmental experiences, personality characteristics) and his or her predisposition for behavior-related health problems: biological dependency (substance abuse), family history (hypertension, obesity), ability to cope (self-efficacy measures), behavior change strategies, and outcome prediction.
2. Interpersonal level. The interpersonal level involves all the social-, family-, and occupation-related relationships of the individual and

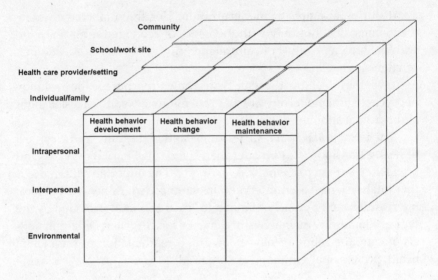

Figure 1–1.   Health enhancement model.
Source.   Adapted from Weiss 1992.

how such relationships may enhance or inhibit health behavior development, change, and maintenance. Social support, peer pressure,
and family environment are seen as reinforcers of behavior throughout the life cycle. Sociocultural influences are included here.

3. Environmental level.   Environmental factors, including the physical setting as well as legal and policy issues, are potent determinants
of health behaviors. These can include access to exercise facilities,
diet, ambient air quality, and statutory regulations. The likelihood of
maintaining individual health behavior change is low in the absence
of environmental modification; programs that focus on the intrapersonal and interpersonal levels without considering concomitant environmental modification are unlikely to achieve the desired
long-term effects.

4. Health behavior development.   The model differentiates among
the processes of health behavior development (brushing teeth, refraining from smoking, prudent dietary habits), health behavior
change, and health maintenance. Development of healthy mental
behaviors (e.g., child-rearing and parenting skills, stress management, planning and coping abilities, very basic mental health education for psychological first aid) can also be considered here.

5. Health behavior change. Health behavior change involves shifting from one set of behaviors to another.
6. Health behavior maintenance. Health behavior and mental health behavior maintenance involves adherence to a healthy behavior, such as a constructive change that has been made, and preventing relapse. Technical approaches to achieving designated objectives in each area may be different. Differences in populations may require strategies tailored to the needs of particular groups.
7. Individual/family. These terms and the ones that follow are self-explanatory.
8. Health care provider/setting.
9. School/work site.
10. Community.

Given the possible "units of treatment" identified in items 7–10, a variety of interventions may be used, ranging from cognitive restructuring to social support and social integration, self-efficacy, social modeling, role models, coping repertoires, positive models, social marketing, communication, community organization, social learning, and community risk reduction. Figure 1–1 maps a 3 X 3 X 4 grid so that there are 36 different areas for consideration, plus a host of possible combinations.

The chapters in this book fall into one or more of these boxes. They begin with individual problems, then move to problems of health care workers, family problems, and problems that involve the whole community. Prevention and health promotion strategies, as well as intervention and health maintenance approaches, are discussed. Many cases present conflicts when people view the problems differently and choose solutions based on different value systems. The psychiatrist can play a useful role in helping to create bridges between these diverse viewpoints and can work with other members of interdisciplinary teams in developing integrated responses.

Intermediate Stages of Health Transition

Looking at Alaska, which is experiencing the middle stages of health transition in an area that falls between very underdeveloped and urban, has many advantages. Processes that are less apparent in urban settings, and are well beyond the resources of less developed countries, can start to be seen and explored. Mental health aspects of the transition process are not well described or understood. In Alaska, however, there are more psychiatrists and mental health professionals than in most developing areas. Village types of problems can thus be looked at in greater depth than they could in most places.

From a public health point of view, if we can learn more about the stages in the transition process, we may find ways to help other groups that are facing increasing contact with the modern industrialized world cushion the blows and minimize some of the social fallout.

In the large regions of the world that are still relatively undeveloped, local indigenous groups are living traditional lifestyles, but rapid economic development is imminent. In parts of Siberia, for example, isolated reindeer herders still have largely nomadic lifestyles. Russia's economic problems will create tremendous pressure for rapid development of the Siberian oil reserves. What sort of future will the indigenous people face? What will the mental health impacts be? Are there ways to prevent major social disruption and still develop the natural resources? What might be learned from the Alaska experience, where there was a "boom and bust" with many changes for Alaska Natives as the pipeline was installed?

These are the kinds of important questions for psychiatrists that this book explores. Too often such topics are marginalized and considered special cases of limited general interest. The experience of psychiatrists in remote rural Alaska, however, can be a model for exploring problems that will become more apparent in the future, as increasing globalization brings countries and cultures into closer contact and psychiatry seeks to be useful in new contexts.

Group for the Advancement of Psychiatry Therapeutic Care Committee and Rural Alaska

In 1985, members of the Therapeutic Care Committee of the Group for the Advancement of Psychiatry (GAP), together with several officials from the American Psychiatric Association, made a working trip to visit remote communities in rural Alaska. The Therapeutic Care Committee has had a long-standing interest in such topics as how to use allied health workers in mental health programs. The purpose of the trip was to learn about the mental health needs of the "special populations" (Eskimos, Indians, Aleuts) in these communities and to explore ways the national organizations might be helpful. The Headquarters Mental Health Office of the Indian Health Service, in collaboration with its Alaska Area program, organized the visit. Within Alaska, much of the trip was arranged by local Alaska Native tribal health organizations and their advisory boards.

The trip was at times physically difficult. The team traveled to small isolated villages, flying long distances in four-seater or six-seater "bush" airplanes or sometimes traveling by boat up turbulent rivers; most of the communities visited were not accessible by road and were 30 minutes to several hours by plane from the nearest small town. The villages, of 100–500 people, relied on paraprofessionals for most health services because even the regional "hub" towns that back up the villages have limited capabilities.

The trip was also at times psychologically difficult. For consultants who come from urban environments, these small villages can communicate a special sense of isolation. Because they usually have no access by road, the feeling of being cut off from "the lower 48" can be acute. Villagers themselves may not feel isolated, especially because they are increasingly linked by radio and cable television, fax machines, satellite dishes, and other devices with the rest of the world. But they often view itinerant professionals as cut off from village concerns, with limited understanding of their problems or ability to help.

Incongruities were striking in the villages. Consultants saw log cabins and racks of drying animal skins next to prefabricated houses, sled dogs next to the latest high-tech snowmobiles, and videocassette recorders in log cabins with wood stoves and outhouses. These communities are at the far end of the "rurality" spectrum. They are not only physically remote, but they give the outsider an impression of psychological and cultural remoteness.

Many of the problems faced in these areas did not fit the standard range of psychiatric practice and seemed almost overwhelming in scope. Complex, interlocking problems have arisen as these small, culturally different communities tried to adapt to the rapid changes in the world around them. As one village man said, "We've had to go from the Stone Age to the Space Age within one generation!"

There were problems of economic development, as cultures built around subsistence fishing and hunting moved to a cash economy. There were spiritual problems stemming from differences between traditional belief systems and those brought in by missionaries. There were educational system problems, housing problems, sanitation problems, problems of basic communication and transportation, and a host of others. Social problems of alcohol abuse, suicides, and family breakdown were prevalent. In addition, there were questions of how to deliver services in such remote communities, with very limited staff and resources, and questions about research and training.

Another difficulty was posed by the message many local people conveyed, which can be summed up as: "We're tired of all these consultants who fly into the village for a few days and then fly off and never see us again. We call that 'airport technical assistance' and we don't need any more! If you really want to help, why don't you 'adopt' some of our communities, come back as much as you can for the next 5 years or so, and really try to learn about our problems and work with us to fix them?"

A number of committee members made follow-up trips to Alaska, during which they held extensive discussions about how to be most helpful and how to respond to the communities' requests to be "adopted" and taken seriously rather than be the subjects of a one-shot tour. Twenty-six trips were made over a 6-year span, with visits to 25 different communities. Some of these visits were brief, 1-day trips. Others lasted 2–3 weeks; members lived in the villages in family homes and returned repeatedly to the same community to attempt to experience local problems as fully as possible and explore potential solutions. Each of the participating committee members visited a number of different towns, cities, and villages to become generally familiar with the state's varied geographic settings and Native groups. Most also made repeated visits to a particular region to learn about it in greater depth.

By accompanying professionals from Alaska Area Native Health Service Area Division of Behavioral Health on their field visits, and through reading a wealth of documents and publications, the committee members tried to learn about the various areas, the people, and their programs. Their contacts during these visits were with health professionals, administrators, patients, and community residents. Educators, magistrates, police officers, pastors, politicians, economic development specialists, and many others were interviewed to get as full a picture as possible of the health programs. The committee's greatest sense of the Native population's views came from the Alaska Natives who worked in the health programs.

Typically, a committee member visited a clinic or hospital, meeting with caregivers, seeing patients, and consulting about treatment issues, and at the same time becoming aware of a variety of problems and needs and gaining an overall perspective of the region. Caregivers usually welcomed this sort of involvement. Consultative interaction with clinicians seemed to have the potential for improving the quality of care; however, since visits were infrequent, they also highlighted the relative isolation and frustration of clinicians between visits. It was not uncommon in the context of a clinical consultation for specialized teaching to take place, particularly about new or unfamiliar techniques. Concepts might range from antidepressant augmentation to family systems techniques to how to manage difficult schizophrenic or bipolar patients.

On some occasions, the consultant served in a peer quality review capacity to help a clinic meet accountability standards. Retrospective chart reviews increased the consultant's awareness of clinic populations and areas of need, both clinical and educational. Other visits served primarily to familiarize a consultant with a program, a region, or a particular population or type of problem.

Caregivers and administrators were sometimes appreciative of outside attention and enjoyed talking of their program. At other times, the response was "What's this all about? What's in it for me?" Committee members had to work hard to clarify the purpose of the visits and tried to give immediate evaluative feedback and offer constructive suggestions. Many programs were truly innovative and could genuinely be complimented. Learning about them was of definite benefit to the consultants, highlighting the two-way nature of the process, and knowledge of such programs could be naturally shared with other regions subsequently visited.

In some programs in crisis, workers requested assistance; in these instances, consultants carried out a variety of activities. For example, incest and child sexual abuse generated strong concerns in several regions. In one, a consultant held problem-defining and problem-solving workshops with representatives of clinics, schools, churches, and village and tribal councils. Other workshops involved clinic caregivers and Native health workers from satellite villages. Similarly, the topics of suicide prevention, crisis intervention, depression, and substance dependency were addressed at various levels in a region, with follow-up wherever practicable.

Some visits focused on self-help and self-determining activities generally regarded as promoting health and reducing dysfunction. For example, committee members accompanied the coordinator of the Iñupiat Ilitqusiat (Spirit Program) on visits to several villages and took part in meetings encouraging greater Elder Council organization and participation. The Spirit Program promotes traditional cultural values such as respect for elders, knowledge of one's family tree, and avoidance of conflict, using Native grandparents to teach youth in special school and camp programs.

In another setting in the south-central part of Alaska, consultants were impressed with the success of one village's move toward sobriety. One of the consultants worked with Native leaders on developing an educational program that could be shared with other villages. The Native leaders' frustration and their positive response to consultation and support cannot be overstated. Again, follow-through and subsequent contact were crucial for success.

Follow-through was accomplished in a number of ways. Sometimes the committee members developed personal relationships with key people in the region. They tried to stay in touch by telephone or by letter between visits. There seemed to be a greater openness and willingness to contact the consultant when the time between visits or other contacts was relatively short (90 days or less) and when the consultant had been on-site long enough or often enough to become comfortable and familiar.

Although much of the committee's work took place in the hub towns and cities, members also visited the remote villages. This helped sensitize them to what life was really like for the patients they had seen presenting in the clinic. It also helped establish a familiarity with health aides, who play a key role in identifying problems and in providing early interventions, appropriate referrals, and continuing care. These people, along with translators and other village leaders, were essential to the consultants being accepted in any useful way. They are critical to the success of any system of health care for the Native population.

Consultative visits were spread very thin, so at times they seemed minimally effective. One Native professional commented early in the program, "You may ultimately have to move here to accomplish what's needed." Yet, because of the high turnover of local staff, even the community leaders who requested a commitment over time were often not present themselves on a follow-up visit just 6 months later. In addition, local people who did make requests of the consultants sometimes seemed to want a kind of help—in developing additional funding or in dealing with complex social and political problems—that did not fit with how the consultants saw their roles. It was therefore difficult in some cases to know what the local people themselves felt should be done that consultants could help with, and difficult in other cases because the local people wanted types of help the consultants were not sure how to provide.

As a result, the Therapeutic Care Committee members had to keep rethinking basic assumptions about what their consultation should consist of, who the consultees should be, who "owned" certain problems, what practical help could be provided, and what role clinicians should play. This reflects the experience of others who have set out to work in settings that are culturally different from their own, particularly when these are remote rural settings. Practices and beliefs that are largely taken for granted must be reexamined as a result of contacts with people holding quite different assumptions and views.

For example, most psychiatrists consider university-trained specialists a basic foundation of the field, and individuals and agencies are increasingly required to be properly licensed and accredited to deliver mental health services. Insurance reimbursements, grants, and hiring practices of social agencies are all "degree conscious." There are also certain preconceptions about the roles consultants should play.

In remote rural areas such as those the GAP consultants visited, the resources are simply not there, and most likely never will be, to get a sufficient number of highly trained professionals to do the work. The local people, therefore, stressed self-help and use of indigenous healers and paraprofessionals, with extensive use of master's level backup people. Training and professional specialization were not valued in the way the consultants were used to. Whether there should even be a billing system was sometimes in question. Local people had considerable skepticism about the potential helpfulness of outside experts. In some cases, they definitely wanted consultation but had very different assumptions about what the consultation should consist of.

Locals had in many cases a service orientation to a larger community and were focused on trying to deal with social causes of illness and on issues of empowerment, local control, self-determination, and maintaining or rebuilding community cohesiveness. Although some individuals were being seen in clinics by professional specialists, there were also group collective actions (e.g., Spirit Camps, "gatherings," ceremonies) in nonclinical settings (e.g., wilderness camps, people's homes) where much of the work was done by nonspecialists. Basic problems such as jobs, housing, education, and sanitation were higher priorities than psychiatric services. Consultants oriented toward helping local people improve only their professional clinical services tended to be seen as elitist and not really dealing with the core problems.

Many indirect experiences contributed to a degree of "culture shock." In the small villages and hub towns visited, people were part of an interconnected system—including magistrates, legal officials, teachers, religious leaders, and political leaders—that the consultants otherwise would not experience directly. After repeated visits, consultants were able to appreciate what the locals had been trying to communicate from the beginning: Their problems were in fact different from those in urban areas, and "off-the-shelf" approaches that might work elsewhere did not fit. In particular, the embeddedness of clinical problems in social and cultural contexts needed to be understood and dealt with.

Historical Underpinnings of
Mental Health Problems

Historical and contextual factors are important in understanding the case material in this book. Attempts to help remote rural areas often include remarkably little attention to historical developments. Yet knowledge of what has gone before and of long-term dynamic trends can be important in developing programs that work. For example, information about language suppression and the role of the schools and churches, outlined later, suggested ways to develop programs based on terms in local languages for mental health conditions and particular types of school-based as well as "Spirit" (cultural values) programs. Developing general principles and frameworks for a cluster of discrete organizations and groups with different concepts of needs and services requires a broad-based, integrated vision that includes the historical dimension.

The assumption here is that the health of human beings is inextricably bound to their embeddedness in social groups. Society and cultures link an individual's needs to social values, provide continuity and transmission across generations, and provide ordered and organized ways to adapt to change. The family is the primary social unit in which these processes occur, but is itself subject to change as the larger society changes.

Given these assumptions, historical events that might otherwise be taken for granted become significant. The emergence of towns and cities, industrialization, large anonymous groupings that are not kin-based, and technological changes all may alter the pattern of social constraints and relations and create potential strains on every aspect of family life, from early attachment in infancy to parental and other family member roles to the family's ability to provide social and emotional support systems and engage in community networks.

Significant Events in Alaskan History

This brief account sketches selected aspects of Alaska's history that seem to have influenced the types of family dysfunction and related behavioral health problems illustrated in the cases (Fienup-Riordan 1992; Fortuine 1989, 1993; Mohatt et al. 1987).

Before the arrival of non-Natives, more than 75,000 Natives lived in Alaska. These people spoke more than 20 different languages, were adapted to as many ecological niches as Alaska's environment could support, and were divided into several hundred often widely different societies consisting of members of closely related family groups. They did not identify themselves as Alaska Natives; their primary allegiance was to families and tribal groups. Major languages were Tlingit, Athapaskan, Aleut, Iñupiaq, and Yupik (Fienup-Riordan 1992).

Confrontation between Alaska Natives and outsiders began with the arrival of the Russian fur traders in the mid-1700s. Although Russia claimed Alaska, the Russians came primarily to exploit resources rather than to expand their territory. The newcomers had colonialist attitudes, but needed Alaska Natives' help as guides and trappers. Early contacts frequently deteriorated into violence. As time went by, however, peaceful relations generally replaced hostility and suspicion.

Many of the early non-Native arrivals were heavy drinkers—soldiers, whalers, and later those associated with the gold rush in the Nome area. Natives were thus exposed to role models who themselves had substance abuse problems. Alcohol was used by the Russians as part of their trade strategy—a strategy that was never explicitly stated but might be paraphrased as "Get people drunk on vodka and they won't want as much for their furs or fight as hard." Some natives may still be experiencing the aftermath of these policies today, as reflected in their heavy, abusive drinking.

Attempts to assimilate Alaska Natives began in the 1800s. By the end of the century, a dozen Protestant denominations and the Roman Catholic and Russian Orthodox churches had established mission stations throughout the state, converting whole villages (Flanders 1991; Kan 1988; Prucha 1988; Van Stone 1964).

Christian missionaries were not the only ones working to transform Alaska Natives. Following the United States' purchase of Alaska in 1867, the first Organic Act of 1884 provided schooling for Alaska Native children. Separation between church and state was far from clear-cut at that time, and during the late 19th and early 20th centuries, Protestant missionaries worked with the federal government toward the twin goals of "civilizing" and "Christianizing" the aborigines so they could achieve the "Anglo-Saxon frame of mind."

The colonial attitude of the Bureau of Education was explicit. In 1906, the bureau chief proposed teaching Natives "what a white man wants of them, so that the white man can use these men for things that are useful for his civilization" (Fienup-Riordan 1992, p. 5); this statement appears to be representative of attitudes at the time. There were educators who were also missionaries, and religious groups such as the "Society to Reform the Heathen" that worked on projects such as transcribing oral to written languages, composing dictionaries, and establishing church schools. There was intense opposition to the former Russian policy of bilingualism.

One key to Native usefulness in white society was knowledge of the English language, and the Bureau of Education zealously promoted instruction in English. The superior status of English as "the language of civilization" was assumed. Its exclusive use in government and missionary schools, often harshly enforced, was a direct and intentional assault on Native identity. Even today, although there have been some efforts at bilingual education, many older people recount vivid stories of being slapped with a ruler or made to stand in a corner or having their mouths taped if they spoke their native languages in school as late as the 1960s.

The impact of teachers, like that of missionaries, was not restricted to the classroom. Under their direction, the people built new houses and gained access to an unprecedented array of trade goods and new technological developments. However, although Alaska Natives increasingly spoke English, lived within four walls, worked for wages, and attended school and church, they remained independent; their lives focused on extended family relations and the pursuit of traditional subsistence activities.

Economic developments such as commercial whaling, gold mining, and reindeer herding caused additional disruptive impacts. In the 20th century, the arrival of military personnel and attendant service industries during World War II brought a non-Native population that was for the first time as large as the Native population. Although some Alaska

Natives served in the armed forces, most remained quite cut off. Native people in the military were not only exposed to the wider world but also to greater use of alcohol as an aspect of socialization into military culture.

By the time Alaska became a state in 1959, the relative lack of commercial resources and the geographic isolation of many Native communities had reduced contacts with and innovations from the outside world. Village economies were depressed. The push for statehood came mostly from non-Natives, who wanted greater control of the state's natural resources to help deal with the economic decline.

In the 1960s, the "War on Poverty" sought to diminish the widening economic gap between Alaska Natives and the non-Native society. State and federal agencies advocated economic development in rural Alaska to allow Alaska Natives to make the transition from their subsistence existence to a more self-supporting one with adequate income and employment. The continuing implication was that Alaska Natives should strive toward the goal of non-Native society.

After statehood, Alaska Natives mobilized to protect their land interests and to address their social needs. Reacting to land selections by the new state government, Native organizations made land claims throughout Alaska. Those claims remained unresolved until it became clear that oil fields, discovered on Alaska's North Slope 10 years after statehood, could not be developed until the Native claims were settled. In 1971, Congress passed the Alaska Native Claims Settlement Act (ANCSA), which awarded Alaska Natives 44 million acres and $1 billion and called for establishment of corporations to manage those assets. Tremendous wealth came to the state as the oil resources were developed, but the boom was followed by a bust after the Alaska pipeline was completed. The development of oil production led to increasing minority status for Alaska Natives with the substantial influx of non-Natives. Currently, only about 16% of the state's population is Alaska Native.

Health and Mental Health History

Associated with these historical developments, there have been major changes in the population's health conditions and in the available service system. In his book, *Chills and Fever: Health and Disease in the Early History of Alaska,* Fortuine (1989) provided a good summary of many of these.

The 19th century was characterized by tremendous population disruption for Alaska Natives. Communicable disease, such as the smallpox epidemic of the 1830s, wiped out whole villages. Subsequent epidemics in the 1900s of influenza and tuberculosis also took a tremendous toll, undermining leadership, damaging personal relations, and leading to major population declines.

The 20th century saw a shift in leading causes of mortality from infectious disease to "behavioral lifestyle" disease (e.g., alcoholism, domestic violence, suicides, child abuse). In the 1990s, about half the population of 87,500 was under age 16. This younger group has substantial problems associated with fetal alcohol syndrome, child abuse, childhood obesity, childhood use of smokeless tobacco, childhood inhalant abuse, and high rates of teenage substance abuse and suicidal behavior. Many social problems, such as the inadequate educational system and lack of economic opportunities, continue today as they have in the past. As the population of children with problems grows older, increasing strain on the existing tertiary care system is expected, unless effective prevention and early intervention strategies can be developed.

Social and Family Changes

Among Native families, there have been trends toward: 1) single-parent families headed by Native mothers (this is in part a response to welfare policies that give a woman financial aid if she is unmarried with children, but expect the husband to provide financial support if a couple is legally married); 2) interracial marriages (more Native women marry non-Natives each year than marry Natives); and 3) unmarried Native males (Mohatt et al. 1987).

Families, especially in rural areas, are still fairly large, with 27% living in households of six or more people. The population is young, with about two-thirds of the Native population under age 30 and about 3,500 new babies per year. The population is growing at about 3% per year, creating an increasing strain on child-related services that were already swamped and are now experiencing cutbacks.

As one example of how changes in family structure present, one rural region of the state has about 200 births per year to Native women. In a recent year, 40 births were to teenage mothers; of these, only 3 were reported by marriage certificate data to be married. Many had dropped out of school and so are at risk as single, teenage, relatively uneducated parents. Of the older Native women, about 60% of those who did marry had non-Native spouses. This represents a tremendous "flight of the female" away from traditional Native family roles for women.

Prenatal care and neonatal mortality for this group are surprisingly good, reflecting active efforts to educate women, encourage prenatal care, and treat high-risk pregnancies in hospital settings rather than using village midwives. Once the infants go home, however, mortality rates rise considerably. This is felt to reflect social and behavioral pathology in the homes (e.g., parental alcohol abuse leading to inadequate child care, childhood injuries, child abuse). The focus in the past has been on interventions such as well-baby clinics and immunizations. Studies on traditional concepts of child rearing, and on ways to reinstitute social and cultural practices that might strengthen family values, are just beginning.

Many Alaska Native men are unprepared to work in a cash economy and continue with subsistence hunting and fishing or seasonal work. The female-to-male employment ratio for Natives is greater than for non-Natives in all categories except farming, forestry, and fishing. The women's greater access to income also creates a strain on family relations; there are historical roots to this trend (Mohatt et al. 1987).

Families and individuals, embedded as they are within social systems, have been affected in many other ways that influence health behaviors. It is important to remember that many of the changes in the social system and associated disruptions in families resulted from well-meaning attempts to be helpful. The churches, the educational programs, and the government efforts to provide new organizational structures and aid to families with dependent children all were seen at the time as improvements. Corporations formed under the ANCSA were intended to improve local control and self-determination and to safeguard the interests of future generations.

The values of the "helpers," however, tended to promote individualism: personal salvation through religious conversion, rights of individual shareholders to stock in the new corporations, and ideas about personal property built into legal rulings concerning land transfers and money settlements. Over time, this appears to have weakened collective identity and traditional community and family values, giving rise to behavioral problems that are now often identified as conditions that psychiatrists and other mental health professionals should somehow fix.

Structure of Rural Health Care

Regional health corporations, formed in 1971, have assumed increasing responsibility over the years in managing regional health organizations in Alaska. Typically they serve a number of villages, supervising village health workers, village clinics, and paraprofessionals working on mental health and substance abuse problems. Emergency medical staff and itinerant public health nurses are available in some bigger communities. There are, however, more than 200 small villages, ranging in size from 100 to 500 people, often an hour or more away from the nearest regional hub town.

In the regional town, which may have a population of 5,000–10,000, there is often a small general hospital of 12–35 beds, staffed by family physicians, nurses, and social workers. Mental health and substance abuse services may be available to a limited degree in the town. Villagers must be flown into town by charter plane to access these services; telephone backup systems allow the village health workers to call the regional staff to decide whether the patient should be flown in.

The relatively small regional budgets come largely from state grants and federal contracts, which have not been rising to keep pace with inflation. Staffing and facilities are meager, and the costs of delivering care are high. Programs are, therefore, usually underfunded, given the scope and complexity of the problems with which they are faced. (Legal battles have been going on for many years over "mental health lands," set aside at the time of statehood. Revenues from these lands, which were supposed to provide mental health program funding, have been used for other purposes.)

At the village level, most services are provided by village health aides with, in some cases, village paraprofessional alcohol and mental health counselors (Caldera 1988; Caldera et al. 1991; D'Augelli 1982; Quick and Bashshur 1991). There is a certification system, an extensive training manual, and a *Village Drug Reference*, which is like the *Physicians' Desk Reference* but with a simplified formulary of drugs that can be given locally with telephone backup from the regional family physicians (Preston et al. 1992). Training materials for local village response teams, which include the health aide, other counselors, the safety officer (like a paraprofessional village police officer), school counselors, and others, are also being developed. The idea of the team training is partly to diffuse responsibility because many villagers are related to each other. In addition, when one of the counselors is out of the village, the cross-training allows someone else to cover. Urban centers, where psychiatrists are available and facilities are better, are often 1–4 hours away by plane. Travel to the remote rural areas can be expensive, both in money and time; flights are often canceled because of weather.

Problems and Challenges in
Remote Rural Alaska

Some of the challenges for psychiatrists working in remote rural Alaska result from the enormous size and the widely scattered population of the state. Figure 1–2 shows Alaska's land area compared with the rest of the United States. As can be seen, a person on the end of the Aleutian Chain may be 4 hours or so by plane from the nearest hospital, located in the center of the state in Anchorage. This would be similar to a patient flying from Los Angeles, California, to Boston, Massachusetts, for general hospital care.

Figure 1–3 shows the distribution of Alaskan communities by location and population level. More than 200 communities, many with fewer than 800 residents, are widely scattered geographically; to reach them

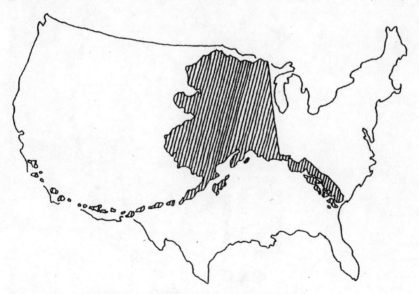

Figure 1–2. Alaska: size comparison with "the lower 48."

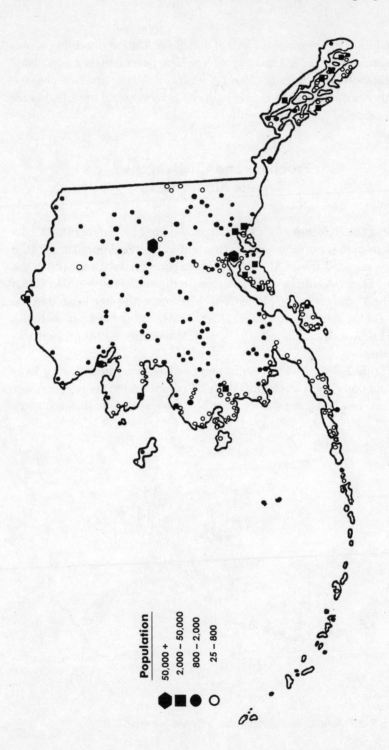

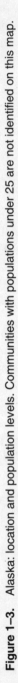

Figure 1–3. Alaska: location and population levels. Communities with populations under 25 are not identified on this map.

entails major costs in airplane fares and staff time.

Only about 19 of these communities have road access. As shown in Figure 1–4, the rest can be reached only by boat, by plane, or sometimes by snow-machine or dogsled. Some types of treatment, such as group therapy, are nearly impossible; a village may have only one or two people who could benefit, and assembling a bigger group is too expensive and complex.

The multiple cultural groups and languages in Alaska are shown in Figure 1–5. Within each region there is great diversity not only of cultures and languages, but of ecology, history, local economy, degree of culture contact, educational levels of the population, and so on. This makes standardization of programs very difficult. They must be tailor-made for each specific location, because the regions tend to be at different organizational levels and to have a different mix of local capacities and resources.

Within many of the regional programs, some villages have felt that their unique problems were not addressed, even with regionalized programming. In recent years, a number of villages and subregional groups have requested independent state and federal grants so they can manage their own village-based programs. Not surprisingly, this leads to even greater complexity; new organizations with little experience in managing health programs all request technical assistance and medical and psychiatric backup. As programming is increasingly localized, the tendency is to find more cases; this puts a strain on the regional and urban programs, which must provide increased amounts of specialized care, but which have to share regional funding with the new village programs.

Table 1–1 highlights some differences between urban and rural models of care. The dichotomy is somewhat artificial: some locations in big cities are severely underserved and have some of the characteristics shown in the rural column, whereas some rural areas are relatively well-off. In the kinds of remote rural and developing locations discussed in this book, however, the differences from even the poorest urban ghetto are marked. Cities, if nothing else, have much better transportation and communication systems; access to specialists and to technology is considerably easier than in extremely isolated situations.

Other challenges faced by mental health professionals in remote rural areas become apparent over time. Change takes place slowly in remote rural programs, and complex social forces are involved; workers feel less instrumental in bringing about change and less certain of their

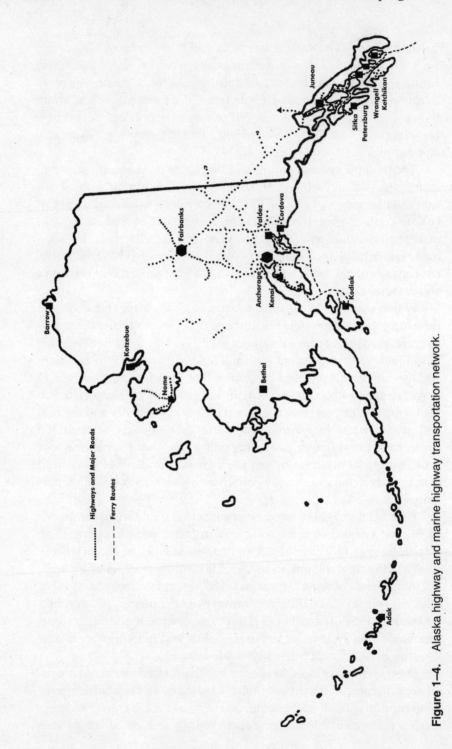

Figure 1–4. Alaska highway and marine highway transportation network.

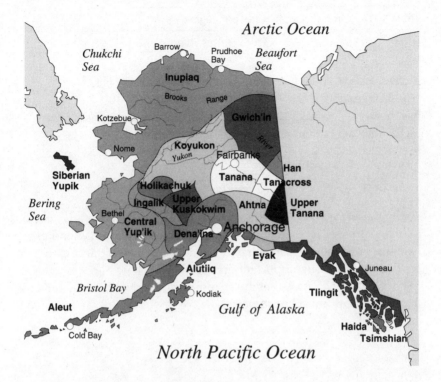

Figure 1–5. Language groups of Alaska.

own contribution to final outcomes. In small communities, the interconnections between mental health problems and individuals in the family and wider community are readily apparent, making workers sometimes feel overwhelmed or "stuck." A major challenge is to help therapists acquire more sense of "maneuverability" and patience in dealing with enmeshed, long-standing, chronic problems.

At present, Alaska's population has many health problems related to unhealthy lifestyles—substance abuse problems in particular, but also problems resulting from changes in nutrition, family violence, suicides, and so on. The service system is increasingly managed by Alaska Natives directly, in a spirit of self-determination. It is tremendously difficult, however, to provide access to care in remote, widely scattered, small communities whose population is heavily weighted toward young people.

The health system, originally set up to deal with infectious disease

Table 1–1.   "Urban" versus "rural" paradigms

Urban	Rural village
Specialists	Generalists
Professionals	Paraprofessionals; self-help
High technology	Low technology
Individuals	Extended families; communal systems
Higher standard of care	Lower standard of care
Individuals with insurance	Low, fixed budgets for population that is mostly "uninsurable"

epidemics and acute-care health problems, is making major adaptations to deal with the large number of people with chronic behavioral problems requiring long-term rehabilitation. Even if better access to care could be worked out, important questions about how to respond effectively when health problems are so interconnected with social and economic problems must be answered.

A Global View

The health problems of the developing world are already overtaxing limited national expenditures, and problems associated with the newly emerging chronic diseases will have to wait until more pressing issues are brought under control. These issues include clean air and water, sanitation and waste disposal, control of infectious disease vectors, immunization, maternal and child health, and preventable injuries—health problems very similar to those faced a century or two ago by the now-industrialized countries. Remote rural areas in the developed countries have some of the same problems.

It is difficult in subsistence economies to gather sufficient resources to improve the health of the population. Given these limited resources, improvements in the health status of a population are unlikely to come from the more expensive "curative" side of health care technology.

Presenting interventions in a socially and culturally acceptable form, getting people to adopt the necessary changes as their own, and building the infrastructure necessary to sustain these changes all require collaborative efforts from many disciplines integrated within a common conceptual framework. Participants may include epidemiologists to look at patterns of disease incidence and prevalence, anthropologists and sociologists to explore the cultural and social contexts, psychologists and psychiatrists to evaluate objective and perceptual issues from the standpoint of the individual as well as biologists, physicians, physiologists, geneticists, and biostatisticians. Each participant works at a different level of analysis to improve overall understanding of a multifaceted health problem.

Fighting Malaria in the Amazon

The following vignette, from a discipline seemingly far removed from psychiatry, provides an especially striking example of the failure of what specialists first pinned their hopes to—a strictly biomedical cure for malaria problems in remote areas of Brazil. It also illustrates the kinds of prevention and disease elimination programs that can be possible when social science approaches are combined with biomedical ones and multiple disciplines make multiple levels of analysis possible (Sawyer and Sawyer 1992).

After national control activities began in Brazil in the 1940s, malaria decreased from an estimated 6 million cases per year (one-seventh of the population) in 85% of the municipalities to 52,469 officially reported cases in 1970; of these, 72% were in the Amazon. It looked as if the problem was on its way to being eliminated and was contained largely in one region of Brazil.

The number of cases has grown steadily ever since, however, with 560,143 cases in 1990 and a million expected in coming years. Conventional technological approaches, including house spraying with DDT, case detection with blood slides, and the distribution of antimalarial drugs, were no longer working.

The problem seemed to be that "frontier malaria" in the Amazon had different characteristics from the "stable malaria" in more urbanized parts of the country. There was high vector density because of the large number of mosquitoes and intense exposure to vectors in the damp rain forests, with significant outdoor transmission. Migrants common in the region had low levels of immunity and limited knowledge of the disease. Morbidity was high and fatality relatively low; there were many people who could be sources of infection. Drug-resistant strains of falciparum malaria were also increasingly frequent.

The difficulty of applying conventional control measures was exacerbated by weak presence of other institutions, little sense of community, and high population mobility, as well as political marginality. Reversal of the former downward trend in rates of malaria was therefore attributed in part to technical factors, such as resistance to insecticides and drugs, but mainly to social, economic, demographic, and environmental forces. Preventive and curative health activities appeared to be at odds with ecological and socioeconomic factors—methods of clearing the forests, sanitation, mobility of settlers, housing, transportation, communication, and immunity.

In addition, the design of the malaria prevention program was not entirely appropriate for the frontier areas. Long distances, the warm and humid climate, dense vegetation, high vector density, inadequate roads and transportation infrastructure, the newness of the settlements, the mobility of the population, and the lack of qualified personnel all interfered with its implementation. Over the years, however, DDT and chloroquine had turned out to be effective "researchicides," making it seem unnecessary to devote much attention to a disease on its way to eradication.

A multidisciplinary research team was formed, including economists, demographers, sociologists, architects, political scientists, and parasitologists, to investigate the reasons for rising malaria rates at the individual, family, community, and environmental levels. Their surveys and analysis led to development of low technology, self-help control emphasizing the participation of the settlers themselves: building houses farther away from water, screening doors and windows, making wider clearings around houses, refraining from planting permanent crops near houses, draining and filling (or oiling) breeding places, facilitating the flow of water in streams, avoiding unnecessary contact with the forest and with water, staying indoors after dusk, and using various protective approaches (e.g., bed nets, coils, sprays, repellents, protective clothing). These solutions involved mobilization of communities to make major lifestyle changes. The result is that malaria in this region once again seems to be on the decline.

From a psychiatric point of view, many difficulties similar to those faced by the malariologists block standard types of mental health interventions from working. In the future, psychiatrists may also participate in multidisciplinary teams that are much broader based than those of the past, involving demographers, epidemiologists, anthropologists, and others in tackling difficult remote rural mental health problems.

Underlying Questions of the Case Studies

Several questions form the basis of the approach to the cases in this book and provide a framework for examining the problems and discussing possible solutions.

How Can the Case Be Viewed in the Context of the Community?

This first question states the underlying theme of the book. The situations presented, even those that seem to concern isolated individual patients, all involve multiple potential service providers and even facilities and often deal with a "snapshot," at a single point in time, of what is really a dynamic series of events with many different aspects.

The networks of relationships to be assessed, as potential forces affecting the treatment plan and as possible resources, can include the standard ones assessed in work with individuals or with family systems and some additional ones that are not so standard. For example, in assessing a family in a city, the psychiatrist would not usually have to consider the impacts of some larger community on every aspect of the treatment plan, and the impacts of a still larger community on the other two. For a family seen in a village, however, it would be routine to factor in the resources and backup capacity available in the regional hub town and to consider what specialized help from larger cities could be brought to the regional center to back *it* up.

Similarly, plans for rehabilitation of a patient in a village will have to include factors such as the local economy. If 70% of the people in that particular village are out of work, standard vocational rehabilitation efforts for a chronic mentally ill patient may encounter difficulties without highly specialized job coaching and other resources that may not be available and may have to include a plan to deal with the reactions of other, out-of-work villagers if the patient succeeds in getting work.

Looking at the community context also means considering questions of "volume." Most psychiatrists are trained to assess and respond to an individual patient or family or small group. In remote rural areas, however, there may be large numbers of people in the population with similar conditions. From a public health point of view, the question becomes, "What if there are 100 or 200 cases like this instead of just one—what sort of services need to be developed?"

The health and mental health enhancement model outlined earlier (Figure 1–1) provides a framework for considering what factors are initiating and maintaining the health problems described in the cases and what might be done at various levels to assess further and to intervene.

Who "Owns" the Problem?

A second underlying question in each case is, "Who 'owns' the problem?" In remote rural areas, multiple public agencies are often involved, with overlapping jurisdictions and responsibilities. There are also very real issues of empowerment and of how best to prevent undue dependency on scarce professional resources.

What Can Be Done for the Immediate Problem?

This third question tends to be the initial focus of most clinicians and of most people involved in any case. In remote rural areas, there is often tremendous pressure from local people to fix problems immediately, and usually some person or difficulty is selected as "the problem."

Mental health professionals in these areas need to anticipate this question and provide a list of possible stopgap measures that have been partially successful elsewhere. The psychiatrist who travels to a variety of isolated rural communities soon collects information on successful approaches and often can serve a useful function by passing on ideas from one community to another.

What Else Could Be Done?

Better results are often achieved by solutions that are not so obvious and time driven, which prompts the fourth question, "What else could be done?" Stepping aside from the immediate problem allows an approach that addresses the underlying issues that led to the problem in the first place. Rather than only "putting out fires," building preventive basic capacities so the "fires" will not occur is encouraged. (The "capacities" being built include abilities to do planning, staffing, organizing, budgeting, evaluating as well as implementing of programs directly by the local people.) Considering the total health needs of the community, and not simply the care of an individual patient, may require broad-based community development and local capacity-building approaches.

When resources are limited, however, an "ounce of prevention" may be all that is available, even if a "pound of cure" would be preferable. A framework such as the health enhancement model in Figure 1–1 is helpful in looking systematically at a wide variety of possible health enhancement strategies.

Many of the possible solutions discussed in the cases involve extensive community education and efforts to change community norms about the acceptability of unhealthy lifestyles. A "marketing" of social health ideas can be involved. There is also an emphasis on development of registry systems and applied epidemiology projects, as well as on setting up early case-finding systems for at-risk populations. Training of local teams is stressed, along with support of the primary care system, including local family physicians, counselors, and paraprofessionals.

Longer-term solutions that will leverage scarce resources and multiply their impact are encouraged. Switching "levels" is often a possibility—a problem difficult to solve at the village level might respond to a regional or statewide effort. Alternate "systems" are also discussed—a problem that is not resolved by working through the health system may be easier to deal with through the school system, economic development, or some other approach. Unfortunately, these approaches are not emphasized in most training programs.

What Should the Psychiatrist's Role Be?

This final question is important to psychiatrists and the community. Some problems in remote rural areas may seem overwhelming at first, particularly for psychiatrists who see their role as a "Lone Ranger" who single-handedly solves the problem. In some situations, the psychiatrist's job may be to identify other people who may more appropriately be involved; in others, a multidisciplinary team effort may be required.

In isolated rural settings, roles are often blurred; a specialist may be asked to do all sorts of things that are not initially expected to be part of the job. Being clear about limits, but flexible enough to adapt to local needs and provide relevant services, takes constant awareness and negotiation.

Training issues may also surface as the psychiatrist begins to consider who else should be involved, or could be involved if training were provided. Psychiatrists themselves may find they need training—for example, a psychiatrist trained as a clinician may have to acquire skills in curriculum design if suddenly called on to design a training program for paraprofessionals.

Psychiatrists who work in remote rural and developing areas will find the questions underlying the case studies in this book useful in thinking about their own work and valuable as a basis for discussion and cooperation with their colleagues.

2

Case 1: Dog Bone

The case presented in this chapter illustrates, among other things, some of the family burden experienced when gravely disabled mentally ill patients from small, remote communities prove uncommittable, and local resources to provide alternative care are virtually nonexistent (Bachrach 1977, 1982, 1983; Barton 1992; Bisbee 1982; Jones 1985). It also illustrates the multiple organizations and service providers that may be involved in such a case, sometimes seemingly working at cross-purposes. Psychiatrists and other mental health professionals in these situations really have their work cut out for them, because although a host of agencies and categorical programs may be involved, there is often only a minimal overall system, and treatment resources that cities and larger rural communities might take for granted are frequently lacking. Family members and health care providers may just give up and abandon the patient, leaving the psychiatrist and others who do get involved with a difficult set of problems. Because resources are not in place, the treatment strategy needs to include some "system building."

The patient is a 30-year-old single, unemployed man with an 11th-grade education. He lives in a village of 100 people, about 30 minutes by charter plane from the nearest rural town (population 2,000). The nearest public psychiatric hospital is another 3 hours by plane from the town.

The village has a small health clinic, staffed by a paraprofessional village health aide. She is a woman born and raised in the village, about 45 years old, who has successfully brought up a large family and who is now a grandmother. She has the equivalent of a fourth-grade education and has had about 75 hours of training in "basic health" but feels much more comfortable dealing with physical problems than with psychiatric ones. In addition, she is a relative of the patient, as is common in a small village where most people are related to each other.

She approaches the psychiatrist who is visiting the village for the first time in several years. He is there only because bad weather conditions forced the charter plane he was in to set down; he has come to the clinic to try to be of some use while waiting for a change in the weather.

The notes in the clinic chart are extremely brief. From a combination of records review and discussions with the health aide, the psychiatrist is able to reconstruct the patient's story.

About 12 years ago, when the patient was 18, he came into the clinic. He said he "ate salad and pig meat at the school, got congested, and has been sick ever since." He cited quotes from the Bible and spoke of evil spirits in people. Since then he has come to the clinic many times with complaints of lung disease secondary to "swallowing asbestos" and with fears of venereal disease, of exposure to radiation, and most recently of acquired immunodeficiency syndrome (AIDS).

A persistent complaint has been that he was damaged by swallowing a dog bone. He clutches at his throat constantly, changing his voice tone. He is described as walking around the village talking "weird"— sometimes making sounds like a dog, at other times high-pitched sounds like a chicken. When asked about this, he says he swallowed a dog bone as a child and then swallowed asbestos when he was 10.

He lives with his parents at their home. He is the oldest of five children, most of whom live nearby. He occasionally is "provoked" by family members and reacts by pushing and kicking them. On several occasions, the village public safety officer (VPSO) has held him briefly in the village jail for assault and battery. (The VPSO, like the health aide, is a paraprofessional; he handles problems in the village that would be handled by police in big cities. For serious crimes, a state trooper can be called in from the regional center, provided that weather allows flights to get in.) In this case, the VPSO, a young man in his early 30s who just recently started his job, is the patient's second cousin. When asked about the pushing and kicking incidents, the patient states, "Our number one problem is that people are evil. They act like they are not the evil ones, even though it is they who are evil."

About 3 years ago, his mother came to the village clinic. She declared that "He's not too much of a problem at home right now. He's been complaining for a number of years about health problems and worries about everything, especially that his brothers and sisters don't know about God. He spends most of his time reading the Bible. The main problem comes when he starts thinking we're evil and threatens us or gets violent and tries to beat us."

Many attempts were made to get him to come to the clinic, but he refused. A family physician on a field clinic visit thought thiothixene might help, but the patient refused any medications. The village health aide was supposed to follow up, but the patient never kept appointments.

A year later, the parents came to the clinic; the patient's threats had increased, and they feared he might be dangerous. A social worker visiting the village went over to the house to see if the patient would talk. "He gave me a push and told me to get out." His parents were instructed in procedures for commitment if he got more dangerous. However, the parents knewof other people from the community who had been committed and then rapidly discharged; on return, these patients were often angry at having been committed and seemed even more dangerous. Therefore, the parents were reluctant to push for involuntary commitment.

Several months later his mother suggested he might go into the city for a checkup. The patient got angry and threw things at her while clutching at his throat and making barking sounds. She was afraid to go home, but finally went back to the house with her husband.

Attempts to get him to go to the rural town for psychiatric clinics have been unsuccessful. He says he has a fear of flying. "I'd just like to get a girl and take off with her and live in peace, but people would come and destroy our peaceful relationship. I don't need a medical checkup."

A year later, the patient was brought into the rural town by the state trooper. He had attacked one of his younger brothers and was charged with fourth-degree assault. He appeared to be rambling and free associating. "Papers were taken from me in 1982 by mobsters and prostitutes. It was evidence on children that were murdered. I'm going to get headhunters to track them down." He kept putting his hands on his throat and changing his voice while speaking like a chicken.

There was now a question of whether the patient was competent to stand trial; he didn't seem to understand that he would be tried on the assault charge. He told the public defender that he had been a prosecutor and a juror himself and said that the public defender was corrupt. During this interview he acted inappropriately, sticking his fingers in his sneakers, putting his hand over his nose, and pressing his hand against his throat.

He didn't want any medications. "I'll take coffee, aspirin, and my mother's nitroglycerine pills to feel better." He also said he had no money to buy food and was living at home on a diet of coffee, plus a flour, sugar, and water mixture. He said he was "going illiterate" because he hadn't read or worked in 6 years. His main problem, he felt, was that he had been shot in the head with a bullet, which had gone right through and left an invisible scar.

At this point the decision was made in the rural town to drop the assault charges and instead try for an involuntary psychiatric commitment. The state statutes allow for commitment if the patient is mentally ill and either a danger to self or others or else "gravely disabled." The commitment papers were filled out, alleging that the patient was gravely disabled and possibly a danger to himself or others. "He does not dress appropriately. He wears only a thin jacket when it is 40–50 degrees below zero outside. People in his village are worried he'll get frostbitten or hypothermia. He walks the beach at night alone in his village, with no place to stay. His parents are scared of him, and he keeps threatening to hurt them and to get revenge if they try to commit him."

He was sent to the city psychiatric hospital, 3.5 hours by plane from his village, but was held for only 3 days. He refused treatment, so there was a commitment hearing. The judge agreed he was disorganized and rambling, not appropriately dressed, and clutching his throat and making odd sounds during the court appearance. The judge did not find him "gravely disabled" or an "imminent danger to himself or others," however, so the judge ordered him released.

The patient signed the discharge-against-medical-advice form and was given a discharge diagnosis of "schizophreniform disorder." Prognosis was felt to be poor because he refused all psychiatric care, including medicines. Only a very brief workup had been done. He refused to return home, saying he intended to go to a shelter in the city. However, he never showed up at the shelter. The parents left the village and got jobs in other communities. They were afraid that he might be violent if he returned home.

The patient apparently stayed in the city about 4 months. He has now returned to the village and is staying alone at his parents' former house. He refuses to come in for evaluations or counseling at the village clinic. People in the village are becoming increasingly concerned, but feel helpless and unsure of what to do next. The psychiatrist wonders how many more people like this live in the surrounding villages, which also get visits from psychiatrists only once every few years.

Mental Health Resources in Remote Rural Areas

Most rural chronically ill patients live with their families, often creating a considerable strain. It is not uncommon in rural Alaska, as happened in this case, for the family eventually to give up and move out, leaving the patient behind in their former house. Local community services for such patients may be almost nonexistent.

Community and family members often show a surprising amount of tolerance for eccentric behavior, up to a certain point. However, once that threshold is reached, often when there is threatening or suicidal behavior, there can be tremendous pressure to eject the patient from the community and great resistance to the patient's early return from an institution.

In urban and rural communities alike, the result of deinstitutionalization policies for chronically mentally ill patients, and noninstitutionalization policies for young chronic patients, has been that many patients get inadequate mental health services (Bachrach 1977, 1982; Jones and Parlour 1985).

In rural communities, limited service structures combine with problems caused by poverty, geographic isolation, lack of transportation, conservative attitudes, and sparse population to produce formidable barriers to effective service delivery. Furthermore, in rural communities, services tend to be geographically dispersed, if available at all, with each agency having its own funding and service eligibility requirements. No comprehensive system exists whose purpose is to identify a client's needs and to respond appropriately.

Available resources can be grouped into three overlapping categories, or sectors: 1) the popular sector, consisting of families, members of social networks, and patients themselves; 2) the folk sector, consisting of traditional healers; and 3) the professional sector, consisting of practitioners of biomedicine (Jones and Parlour 1985).

Where access to professionals is limited, sick people tend to rely heavily on themselves, their families, and other members of their social circle for care. Remote rural communities are highly variable: Some have lots of community support and local cohesiveness, as well as traditional healers, whereas others are fragmented and polarized.

Linkage With the Primary Health Care System

Chronically mentally ill patients have increased needs for medical care; they receive treatment for physical disorders twice as often as patients without mental illness (Jones and Parlour 1985). They may also need mental health care, psychopharmacological interventions, monitoring of subsequent progress, help in adjusting to crises, collaboration with community support and rehabilitation programs, and facilitation of their reentry into the community through legal health status certification.

The amount of care family physicians are willing to provide for these patients varies considerably. Many feel both helpless and hopeless in the face of chronic mental illness that cannot be cured. These family physicians, however, can be extremely important.

Traditional medical practice is part of the natural support system in the rural community. Unless a family member has very severe symptoms, rural people prefer to receive all their health care, including mental health care, from primary physicians. The stigma of "craziness" is such a problem that as many as half of those with mental disorders seek no help. The rural ethic is conservative; people are expected to solve problems on their own or with the help of traditional supports, such as family, friends, church, or family doctor. Formal mental health services are alien to this cultural system, and persons in need of mental health care suffer additional hardship when they are seen to receive services from a community mental health center (CMHC) or a psychiatrist.

The integration of rural health and mental health services via linkage at the primary care level is a solution for certain types of problems. The principal advantages are greater accessibility and acceptability; better case finding, referral, and follow-up care; and improved coordination of care. The linkage concept may be extended to include schools, welfare offices, probation offices, jails, hospitals, and other agencies and can involve local social and community supports, paraprofessionals, family members, and even traditional healers. The disadvantage is that the rural medical system tends to have an acute-care medical model, which can be less sensitive to social and community problems and less skilled at rehabilitation of chronic patients.

Lack of Other Support Resources

Families have become the real primary caregivers for a large population of long-term mentally ill persons as deinstitutionalization has progressed. Yet the presence of a chronically ill family member may burden a strained family to the point that supportive functions are impossible without help. Unfortunately, it may be difficult to enlist indigenous volunteer workers. Geographic isolation and transportation problems undermine volunteerism as much as they do access to health care. Education of widely dispersed rural populations about needs for health and mental health services in the community has remained a challenge.

Extended kinship groups and churches are informal support resources that assume responsibility for their own people. Many of those needing mental health services, especially crisis intervention services, are in marginal circumstances in the community, however, and they are unlikely to receive neighborly assistance from family or church. Some fundamentalist churches believe that mental problems are caused by demons and should be handled by spiritual treatments rather than psychiatric ones; therefore, they may not always cooperate with treatment plans. Similarly, rural Alcoholics Anonymous groups are often quite conservative about patients on psychotropic medications, disapproving of these "mind-altering drugs."

Extreme visibility is also a problem. Although urban programs can often use a kind of camouflage to protect patients' identities, this is difficult to accomplish in most rural places. Both the users and the providers of services are highly visible and lack anonymity. Because patient and therapist may meet on social occasions, a single well-defined role relationship is rare.

Identifying Potential Resources

In Dog Bone's case, events have occurred in a village as well as at the regional level and even at the urban level where the state psychiatric hospital is. Many people from various health and legal organizations are involved. In this situation, actions may have one set of consequences locally and a different set of consequences in another part of the system. For example, decisions by a judge in a large city affect villagers in a distant, small community.

Despite these complexities, or perhaps because of them, a useful first step is to identify all the potential resources that might be available to help Dog Bone. Then a more sophisticated social network analysis can be done if necessary.

Table 2–1 illustrates a simple method of identifying all the "players" involved in this case. What initially appears to be a problem of a rather isolated chronically mentally ill patient, living by himself in a remote village, seems quite different after listing everyone who knows about the case and is at least peripherally involved.

The three-level service delivery system includes: 1) a remote location—the village; 2) a rural backup location—the regional hub town; and 3) the urban location where specialists like psychiatrists spend most of their time and where statewide policy is set.

(As outlined in Chapter 1, in a typical Alaska situation, there are a number of small villages of 100–500 people. The region's hub town of 2,000–5,000 people has more services, such as a small general hospital, a regional jail, a few social workers, and possibly a psychologist or a psychiatric nurse. In the urban center, with a population of 40,000–200,000, are specialists such as psychiatrists, as well as some psychiatric beds and other facilities.)

Table 2–1 shows the number of people—at village, regional, and urban levels—who are involved, or who may need to be involved, in solving Dog Bone's problems. It also lists the facilities that may be involved.

Table 2–1. Potential resources for remote rural patients in Alaska

Village	Regional level	Urban level
People		
Patient	Local magistrate Public defender Probation officer	Judge
Village health worker	Psychiatric nurse Traveling public health nurse Family physicians	Psychiatrist/psychologist/ psychiatric social worker State psychiatric hospital staff Planners and policymakers
Family members	Welfare worker	
Village safety officer	State troopers	Department of Corrections staff
Village leaders	Village health worker trainers, regional leaders	Legislators
Facilities		
Village clinic	Small general hospital Small jail	State psychiatric hospital State correctional facility
Local school	Small community college	State university Shelter

About 50 people and seven or eight facilities are potentially "in the loop," and this is a "simple" case.

To amplify the table, costs of various actions could be added. For example, in 1994, the costs of doing an assessment included a 30-minute round-trip charter plane flight from the village to the regional hub town, at $90 for the patient and another $90 for the escort. The 3-hour trip to the urban center was another $450 round-trip airfare for the patient, as well as $450 for the escort. Because of plane connections, the escort had to stay overnight in the city, entailing food and lodging costs. Hotel costs for professionals traveling to the regional hub center from the city were $125 per night. In the village, itinerants who stay overnight would probably sleep in a sleeping bag on the floor of the health clinic, at a cost of $20.

Time and cost factors are important because they influence the practical feasibility of a proposed treatment response. People who should be working closely together may be many miles apart, and their meetings for coordinating treatment plans will be expensive.

Identifying Missing Resources

When charting the people and facilities who are potentially involved in a case, it is also useful to identify those that are missing, because systems building and program development in rural areas frequently involve efforts to add or substitute for missing program elements.

For example, vocational rehabilitation staff to work with patients suffering from difficult chronic mental illness may be lacking, even at the regional level. There may be no neurologist or psychologist in the region. Halfway houses or local mental health beds may be inadequate. If a psychiatric patient needs a structured environment, the local general hospital may have to be persuaded to take the patient until something happens that leads to the patient's arrest and housing at the regional jail; the only other option may be to get the patient admitted to a distant psychiatric facility.

Having identified possible missing resources that would be nice to have, the psychiatrist in a remote rural area may decide to help write grant applications or assist in other ways to get needed services funded. When there are too few patients to justify a certain service, it may be possible to "joint venture" with another service to create some economy of scale. For example, one region developed a combination detoxification unit/homeless shelter. Patients could be detoxified, then move over to the other side of the building and be sheltered while awaiting placement. Savings in staff and facility costs made the program feasible even with relatively small numbers of clients.

Organizing the Available Information

A variety of simple charts, maps, and note-taking techniques can be of great use in both organizing and remembering information. If you are working in a village, or in a hospital, walk it and map it to get to know the physical and social layout of the field site. If you are studying a group that has no physical location (such as a social movement), it pays to spend time "mapping" the social scene (Schatzman and Strauss 1973), charting the relationships among key players. Similarly, it is a good idea to make a kinship chart of a village and to take a census. Of course, remembering all this information is not a problem when there is only one village to work with. With 10 or more at once, however, all with complicated problems, note-taking techniques and memory aids can be quite a help. Moreover, situations tend to repeat themselves in the villages, and an excellent knowledge of available resources and contacts, added to on each visit, is often the key to success.

Bernard (1988) discussed note-taking methods for anthropological fieldwork that can be used by psychiatrists working in remote rural settings. He described methods of building explicit awareness of the little details in life (Spradley 1980) and suggested techniques for keeping notes clear and complete. Bernard also recommended ways to organize field notes, using a laptop computer and a special coding system. Additional information on ethnographic and anthropological frameworks and methods, which can be enormously helpful when adapted to a psychiatric perspective, is discussed in Chapter 9.

Social network assessment.   Social networks can be assessed in terms of their contribution to health and mental health. Factors to consider include the following (Moxley 1989):

1. Size.   The number of people or other social units with whom the client has direct contact, including frequency of contact, mode of contact, and degree of intimacy.

2. Range or composition. The number of different types of people with whom the client interacts (e.g., kin, neighbors, work associates).
3. Density. The degree to which network members know of or have ongoing relationships with each other independent of the client.
4. Dispersion. The location of network members in time and space.
5. Interactional characteristics. The diversity of linkages, degree of social support, duration, intensity, frequency, and so on.

An "eco-map" of the potential resources involved in this case would be a more graphic way of presenting the information in the chart, along with one type of dynamic data (Goodluck 1988; Hartman 1978). Eco-maps display the external aspects of a family's resources; relationships can be represented as positive, cut off, conflicted, close, and so on.

Therapeutic Value of a Good Assessment

Even if the psychiatrist or other mental health professional does nothing else, a good assessment can have many beneficial effects (Helman 1990, 1993; Johnson 1987). People in the community will have the experience of an outside expert asking them how the overall system works, how it might be better organized, and what can be done beyond an immediate quick fix. By paying selective attention to these aspects of the situation, local people may become curious themselves and start looking for ways to link services better and develop new programs. It is difficult to measure this impact, but many gratifying examples could be cited of major turnarounds in small communities that residents attribute to a visit from a psychiatrist or other outside consultant whose questions got them thinking in a new way.

Networks are discussed further in Chapter 6.

Developing Continuity of Care

People with severe psychiatric disorders, such as Dog Bone, need a wide range of treatment and rehabilitation approaches that ideally include (in addition to medication) psychotherapy, family involvement, day treatment, crisis intervention, and brief and extended hospitalizations. They may also need a variety of social services, including housing, financial assistance, vocational training and placement, and medical care. They need case management to promote coordination of services, integration of services across a cluster of organizations, and continuity of care, especially if they have difficulty in locating and negotiating all this assistance themselves.

Continuity of care has two dimensions: cross-sectional and longitudinal. Cross-sectional continuity means that at any given point in the course of treatment, the person is involved in a comprehensive system of care that is appropriately meeting his or her needs. Longitudinal continuity of care means the fulfillment of the person's needs over time.

A dynamic strategy is necessary, therefore, that in the short run focuses on identifying and fulfilling a spectrum of client needs within a complex organizational field and over the long run responds to changing and emerging needs as clients grow, develop, or experience new challenges.

In Dog Bone's case, a village response team was eventually assembled, using the health aide, the VPSO, and a local minister. A regional master's-level person was identified for backup. This person in turn kept in telephone contact with the psychiatrist in the urban center. The village team, after some initial hesitation, went to the village council to discuss the situation with village leaders. They were able to get Dog Bone to go to a family physician at the regional general hospital for a checkup. He was medicated with thiothixene and returned to the village where he is somewhat improved. The village health aide dispenses his medication and checks for side effects and then calls the family physician in the regional town to get advice on any changes in his condition. Brief training for the local village team and the master's-level backup person was provided by teleconference with the psychiatrist.

There is still a long way to go, because most of what would be needed for a comprehensive rehabilitation program is not yet available in this village. In this case, the psychiatrist met with administrators in the Regional Native Health Corporation, outlined the needs, and encouraged them to hire an additional grant writer or to contract for grant-writer services. When this happens, the psychiatrist will help the grant writer with technical aspects of the proposal. If this does not work, further discussions can be held with the village council to encourage them to do more locally, such as getting additional training or possibly their own local programs. Because so many services are lacking in the villages in this region, it appears that the Regional Native Health Corporation, if convinced of the needs, would have the organizational muscle to obtain the necessary funding. The village leaders have taken a step forward in trying to deal with Dog Bone; over time they are expected to advocate for more comprehensive services, at least at the regional town level.

In comparing Dog Bone's case with what might have happened in a big city, it may appear that the situation is overwhelming or that the case was inadequately handled. Compared with what might be possible in a developing country, however, there are a large number of potential resources and forces that can be slowly brought to bear on this and similar problems over a period of years, if the psychiatrist is persistent.

In this and any other case, there is no "right answer." In practice, much depends on the personal relationships that are in place, the experience of the psychiatrist, and the opportunities that may surface in the process of doing the assessment. Psychiatrists are used to asking, "What is the best treatment in my professional judgment?" In remote rural settings, a different question must be asked: "Given the available resources in terms of staff time, travel monies, skill levels, facilities, and a total population to serve, what can be done to begin to work toward 'best treatment'?" Off-the-shelf approaches that work elsewhere may not work here or may need considerable adaptation.

Other Possible Approaches

A range of solutions is being looked at in other rural Alaskan communities. One CMHC, for example, had no standard facilities available to deal with psychiatric crises. A solution was worked out in which the center pays for a week's stay at a local motel for a person in crisis (Barton 1992). The patient is seen daily at the CMHC walk-in clinic, and an on-call staff member is available to the motel owner if there is a problem at night or on weekends. This approach works well for a patient who is being started on antipsychotic or antidepressant medications and who needs to be stabilized before returning home. Overnight stays at the motel are also available to patients once or twice a year for maintenance so they are less likely to go into crisis.

In another community with the same problem, various other facilities (e.g., the general hospital, women's shelter, children's group home, alcoholic treatment center) are paid to reserve a bed or two to be used for a psychiatric emergency whenever the need arises; the

CMHC staff provides backup. This is referred to as a "crisis-center-without-walls" approach.

Families who analyze resources themselves sometimes come up with innovative solutions. For example, parents of a boy with retardation, now in his 20s, wanted him to be able to get a job, having worked for many years to get special education for him and "normalize" him as much as possible. However, the village had widespread unemployment. The family worked with the village council to develop a cottage industry that created new jobs for other community members as well as their son. They came up with this idea after attempting to map out all possible resources that might be used.

Who "Owns" the Problem?

In fee-for-service settings, there may be incentives for finding patients, giving them quality workups and treatment, and then providing follow-up; there may be competition among providers of services. Services in remote rural settings, on the other hand, usually are provided through a mix of paraprofessionals, plus regional public providers who are swamped with huge, difficult caseloads and must respond to a variety of often conflicting and unclear organizational agenda. Patients like Dog Bone, who lack third-party insurance and who resist treatment, are likely to go untreated or to fall through the cracks between various programs with categorical funding. No one is eager to claim responsibility for Dog Bone.

People in smaller communities are not used to the involuntary commitment process, and they may fear that anyone they do commit may soon be deinstitutionalized back home, seeking revenge on whoever reported the situation. In a small community, with only a VPSO for protection, this can be a very real concern.

In this case, mental health professionals made the referral to the legal system, and the judge decided, based on the relatively restricted way the law is written, that the patient is not suitable for involuntary commitment. Thus in some ways the judge owns the problem and will bear some of the responsibility if Dog Bone does assault someone in the village. The situation is ripe for legal-medical wrangling as to who should do what. This, however, does not make the problem go away. The judge is in the city. The patient is in the village, scaring local villagers who want something done and see the situation as a mental health problem rather than a legal one.

Patients Whom No One Wants to "Own"

Dog Bone's threatening behavior and potential for being assaultive make him more difficult for village paraprofessionals and midlevel practitioners to manage than some other types of chronic mentally ill patients. He is just one of a large number of difficult-to-manage patients who create a tremendous family burden as well as a village burden and who are not dealt with easily under current laws with the types of staffing and facilities available in remote rural locations. In this particular region, there are approximately 60 people with very severe mental disorders. These patients are widely scattered, however, so that one village might have one or two and another village a few more. The psychiatrist must think about the best ways to meet the needs of this total population and must also deal with the dispersion factor, which may require village-based programs for 2–5 patients each, rather than one program in a distant center for all 60 patients.

In many cases, chronically mentally ill patients may be drinking or using drugs. Existing commitment laws for involuntary psychiatric patients may restrict commitments of those with substance abuse problems, and alcohol commitment laws may make it hard for patients with severe mental disorders to get the treatment they need.

In many other situations—such as children sniffing gasoline, or sex offenders who are returned from correctional facilities to villages, or persons with medical problems such as deafness plus mental disorders and substance abuse disorders—management at the local level can be extremely difficult, and everyone tends to "pass the buck." Patients who are not dangerous but are scary to others because of eccentric or bizarre behavior, and who are unwilling to accept voluntary treatment, also fall into this category. For example, one patient decided to "prepare for the Olympics" and went into his parents' bedroom each night to do sit-ups and other exercises for hours at a time. He did not want treatment. This was highly annoying and worrisome to the parents, but did not qualify under the commitment laws for involuntary treatment.

Patients who comply poorly with medication regimens create similar problems. They go off their medication, become dangerous, get committed and remedicated, then are sent back home where they soon are off medications again, and the cycle starts all over. This, of course, happens with urban patients as well. The unique aspects in remote rural areas stem from the small numbers of people in the village, mostly interrelated or otherwise connected to the other village residents.

Working out management strategies in the home community for these types of patients, as well as for deinstitutionalized patients, can be extremely challenging. The impact of an individual patient's dysfunction reverberates throughout the village network and can cause considerable distress to many interdependent people. The VPSO or village health worker or some of the key staff at the regional level, for example, may be relatives of the patient; in any case, they certainly are known to the patient and are faced with a difficult problem that affects them personally every day.

What Can Be Done for the Immediate Problem?

A recurring dynamic pattern appears in many cases like Dog Bone's. Each level (village, region, urban center) tends to look to some higher authority at the next organizational level to solve the problem. This can be called a "shifting the burden" dynamic pattern (Senge 1990a). Family members will involve higher-ups in the community. The community members will try to get the patient sent away so that "outsiders" will take care of the problem. Sometimes the outside interveners are able to achieve a temporary fix faster than the locals could; this can prevent the local people from learning how to deal with the problem themselves. Or the outsiders may just pass the problem upstairs to headquarters or a central office.

Intervention at the Local Level

Because of the "shifting the burden" dynamic, village problems tend to be bucked upstairs, or in Dog Bone's case bucked outside to the regional level, and regional problems tend to be sent up the line to the urban or statewide level. One strategy for consultation is to work to reverse this process so that the problems are handled as close to the local level where they started as possible.

This strategy may produce mixed feelings on the part of many of the participants. The principle of returning problems to the lower or village level can be interpreted locally as the higher-ups either failing to address the problem or opting out. The local people may value local control and want to handle many of their own affairs, but they often feel helpless to deal with difficult patients who may also be their relatives. At the village level, many of the standard types of rehabilitation programs, halfway houses, and counseling are lacking. Unless the aftercare program is worked out very carefully, solutions at the village level can easily wind up as a form of "dumping" the patient instead.

To deal with the ambivalence and the practical problems associated with local control, considerable community education may be needed about what is really involved in "community ownership," with encouragement and support for active participation by family and community members in every aspect of treatment planning and program development. Time-limited assistance from outsiders can help the local people develop their own skills, resources, and infrastructure so that they can be more capable in the future. Simple primary care strategies can be designed for implementation by local paraprofessionals with backup from regional family physicians, nurses, and social workers. This means that medication regimens are kept as simple as possible, with a relatively limited formulary, and that self-help and local support groups are encouraged whenever feasible. Whatever is done is ideally carried out in such a way that dependency on outsiders is not reinforced.

Using Less Expensive Solutions

In remote rural areas, limited resources make it vital to look for less expensive solutions to problems whenever possible. This principle means that very difficult decisions must often be made; generally there is a fixed budget and multiple problems all clamoring for solution. Psychiatrists who have paid little attention to funding issues therefore have to learn some additional skills.

When a problem is identified, rural programs often take the initial line that no funding is available; nothing can be done unless the outside expert can find additional funds. In many cases, however, local bookkeepers are poorly trained, and the psychiatrist may discover monies they did not know they had. Cost-sharing and local matching arrangements may be proposed, if the psychiatrist is knowledgeable about how to do this. However, the limitations on available resources are very real, and difficult ethical issues frequently arise, such as what to do when there is not enough money to do the job right.

Within the village, encouragement and support of local possibilities is the first step: self-help and family-centered approaches; local paraprofessionals' efforts; and community involvement in decision making, including active consultation with village health councils, elders (respected older people who are looked to for advice), and indigenous healers. All the potential local resources must work together; otherwise one organization may be trying to strengthen village capacity while others are promoting "traveling cures" (shipping the problem out of town). Networking with the providers at the next level up may be helpful. For example, in the Kodiak region of the state, village response teams are backed up by a regional "multiagency service network." Paraprofessional training and backup systems are all oriented toward getting people to work together and solve the problem as close to home as possible, while holding costs down by maximizing use of paraprofessionals.

Because most professionals are used to an "intervener" role, in which a specialist renders an expert opinion or diagnosis and decides on a treatment plan, they often get caught up in the external intervener dynamic pattern. They come into the village, see the patient, and leave, or have the patient flown in to a regional hub town's clinic. Because this professional care is expensive, visits are made only every 3–6 months or so, and some villages may not get visited at all. Also, this approach tends to leave the family and village resources out of the loop, uncertain of how to cope with returning patients like Dog Bone. Over time, the costs of sending a person out of the community for specialized professional assessments and then back home for deinstitutionalization can be extremely high.

Professionals with experience in remote rural mental health work usually recognize the benefits of building up village capacity and avoiding undercutting local people. When specialized care is needed, active involvement of the locals in every step of the process is attempted. Discharge and aftercare plans are begun when the patient is sent off to a distant specialized facility; otherwise the patient is likely to return home without the local follow-up needed for a good outcome.

Home-Based Approaches and Village Response Teams

At the village level, another option is a home visit to try to convince the patient to comply with treatment or to determine whether to try to commit the patient involuntarily. Who can best do this (e.g., village response team, psychiatrist) should be discussed; a protocol for paraprofessionals to use in making home visits may need to be worked out. The psychiatrist's time may be better used in providing training and backup to the village response team than in doing individual patient assessments. On the other hand, because a home visit provides an opportunity to see 20 or more people in the family network, many of whom may also have problems, it can often be a more valuable use of time than seeing an individual patient in the village clinic. In addition, it can help identify people in the family network who may become "cotherapists" in a low-cost treatment plan.

Medical and Neurological Assessments

Ideally, an assessment of the patient's current medical and neurological, as well as psychiatric, status should be done. In remote rural areas, a neurologist's visit and neuropsychological tests or laboratory tests may require special scheduling. The remote rural psychiatrist therefore must be skilled in basic screening and differential diagnosis to be maximally useful in these settings.

Medication Issues

Since case managers are often not available, and patients in remote rural areas tend to share their medicines with others or to mix medicines with alcohol and other drugs, it is usually wise to keep doses low and medication regimens very simple, especially if paraprofessionals will have to do the follow-up. In addition, because compliance with oral medication is generally poor, local medical and mental health staff often prefer long-acting intramuscular injections for patients who require antipsychotics. Many deinstitutionalized patients, especially young adult chronically mentally ill substance abusers, are difficult to manage any other way.

Support Services

The lack of support services (e.g., vocational rehabilitation, halfway houses) in remote rural settings means that patients wind up either at a distant treatment facility or at home with little to rely on besides self-help, paraprofessionals, and psychotropics (if these are in fact taken as prescribed).

In such cases, a paraprofessional, a relative, or even a volunteer may be recruited to keep up supportive contact with the patient. If medications are used, training about side effects, danger signals, and the backup call system may be needed for the village paraprofessionals and possibly for the midlevel backup people. Practical discussions of how the medicines will get to the village clinic, how refills will be dispensed, and how certain side effects might be handled are also important. In bigger-city programs, much of this might be taken for granted; that is not the case in a small village with only one or two patients of a certain type and staff with minimal training.

Town Meetings

A town meeting that includes village leaders, the VPSO, and the village health worker provides an opportunity to discuss the situation and consider possible responses. Because everyone in the village is likely to be aware of the problem, confidentiality is not usually an issue. A meeting can be advertised in advance, perhaps with a sign posted at the local grocery store or at the health clinic. In a town of 100 people, 10 or 15 concerned people generally show up, including family members, the health aide, people from the school, and tribal leaders.

The itinerant professional who has called the meeting often serves largely as a catalyst and facilitator. Local people are usually open about their concerns and often have good ideas about how better to support the patient. The idea is similar to what has been described by Speck and Attneave (1973) in the family therapy literature as "networking."

The psychiatric consultant needs to be alert for opportunities to call such meetings. Rather than simply seeing the patient (assuming that he or she can be convinced to be seen), it may be equally or more useful to see the local service providers or to have a town meeting in which a variety of participants help develop a treatment response.

What Else Could Be Done?

Often, not much more can be done to solve an immediate problem. The psychiatrist should keep in mind, however, that although a local solution is preferable, there are times when a problem has to be redefined as a regional or statewide one and a solution sought at one of these other levels.

Registry Systems

Setting up a regional registry system for better tracking of chronic mental patients, with ongoing monitoring of medications, might be considered; such a system helps prevent patients from being lost to follow-up in the remote setting. A variety of other special registries for certain types of persons are kept in some regions (e.g., those who have attempted suicide, children who are gasoline sniffers, pregnant women who are substance abusers and at risk for fetal alcohol syndrome children). Unlike private settings, most patients are in a public health system with a single, computerized database; extensive diagnostic and treatment information can be assembled on common clinical problems needing a population-based approach.

Distance-Delivered Education

Regional health aide trainers and community college staff can help provide more training for village paraprofessionals who work with difficult mental patients. This might include developing a mental health telephone backup system, so that village workers can have regular telephone discussions with regional staff about psychiatric patients (Greene and Mullen 1973). Regional midlevel practitioners might use another telephone backup system for regular consultation with the psychiatrist about difficult cases.

Alaska presents a special challenge to cost-effective health education and training. Vast distances, unpredictable weather, and high transportation costs translate into spending of more than $7,000,000 per year by Native health corporations either to send trainers/instructors into the field or to bring employees to a central location for educational purposes.

Long-distance education via satellite is currently being field tested. One hour of Health Link costs $1,500; 250 communities received that hour of instruction at a cost of $6 per village. The pilot programs—on suicide prevention, on life skills for the elderly, and on alcoholism and fetal alcohol syndrome—received a tremendous positive response.

Health aides in a village such as Kasigluk, in West Alaska, are already able to communicate with doctors in Bethel, using computers, modems, and tiny video cameras. Two computers can link over telephone lines and exchange live video images and data, as well as the voice signal. Without the computer connection, health aides have to give information about a patient to a doctor verbally and wait for the doctor to write it down; with it, patient information can be viewed simultaneously by doctor and aide, or the video camera can scan the patient. Further communications breakthroughs are expected to improve dramatically the ability to carry out remote rural psychiatry in the near future.

At the statewide level, epidemiological studies to determine the number of severely mentally ill patients who are behaviorally treatment resistant and advocacy to change commitment laws or admission policies of the state psychiatric facility might be needed. Other problems that could be addressed at the state level include how to detect patients like Dog Bone earlier, how to improve discharge and aftercare planning at the state facility, and how to change third-party financing to encourage more home-based care.

What Should the Psychiatrist's Role Be?

In practice, it is all too easy to fall into a pattern in which local providers define the psychiatrist's role. The psychiatrist then says, "They keep me so busy doing med checks, I don't have time to do anything else," or "I have only 15 minutes to see each patient, so I can't really learn much about him or her—just a brief history and then an attempt at medication based on a cursory workup. This compromises my values and makes poor use of my knowledge."

Such comments indicate that the psychiatrist has allowed the "shifting the burden to the outside intervener" pattern to occur, getting trapped in a narrowly defined role. Local resources that should be involved are not identified; innovative program development to build up missing pieces is not taking place; and a quick-fix approach via medications is in evidence, rather than attempts at fundamental solutions.

Psychiatrists, like other mental health professionals, often are not as skilled at team building and at delegating as they might be. They may often identify a need, then think "But I don't know how to do that," and give up in frustration. The question, "Are there are other people who could work as part of a team on this problem?" seems obvious, but it often does not occur to the psychiatric consultant.

For example, if a local halfway house is needed, a grant proposal must be written to get funding. The remote rural psychiatrist probably is unable to write it. Rather than simply saying, "I don't want to work here with such unsatisfactory services," the psychiatrist can learn to ask who the local grant writers and fund-raisers are and how they might be brought into the process of writing the proposal.

Economic development specialists, religious leaders, educators, and judges may all play key roles and should be considered as potential team members in dealing with particular situations. In considering training problems, the remote rural psychiatrist may work with staff at local community colleges and village schools to develop curriculum and certification systems. Local advocacy systems can help develop political support for building up a program. Affiliations with distant universities and medical schools may facilitate needed research projects.

Considerable improvements in remote rural services can be achieved over time if the remote rural psychiatric consultant can expand his or her role definition to include a more comprehensive view of the job.

An example from the community mental health literature, dealing with "rural" mental health, offers both contrasts and similarities to the Alaska setting. Libo and Griffith (1968) described the communities their team consulted with in New Mexico. They reported on the types of needs assessments they attempted at that time; the historical, demographic, social, political, economic, and cultural attributes of the populations served; and the professional and personal backgrounds of the mental health consultants. They attempted to assess the results of their efforts.

These rural communities had populations of 3,000–7,000, in districts of 12,000–14,650 square miles; district populations were 64,000–103,000. The consultants drove between 15 minutes and 2 hours to reach the communities. This is a very different proposition from Alaska, where communities of 100 people or so, with no road access at all, are scattered over vast territories many times bigger than the whole state of New Mexico. There are many fewer resources to draw on when populations in a district are in the 5,000–8,000 range. The psychiatric consultants described by Libo and Griffith (1968) were able to travel monthly to each location; in Alaska consultants visit every 3–6 months.

Although the issues covered by Libo and Griffith (1968) differ substantially from those considered in this volume, there are also some striking similarities, such as problems in recruiting. The consultants described feelings of personal and professional tension—that they were "snowed under," that the experiences were highly anxiety provoking, that they "never realized how protected" they had been in their past work in hospital and clinic-based settings. (Problems of burnout are discussed in more detail in Chapter 5.)

Another similarity was that measurement of results was not done by standard clinical criteria. As Libo and Griffith (1968) stated, there were "no successes or failures." The projects' results were looked at in terms of community responsiveness and readiness to make changes. Cases similar to Dog Bone's, which might be seen by psychiatric residents as minimally successful, actually included a whole portfolio of intervention strategies to build up local capacity and a service system using village response teams, backup systems, and so on. From one standpoint, Dog Bone, like many other chronically mentally ill patients, is still not doing too well. From another point of view, however, found both in Libo and Griffith's (1968) book and in this volume, an approach is evolving that should, in the long term, lead to improved options for local community-based care.

Example From Another Setting

Mental Health in Africa

German (1987) provided an overview of mental health problems in Africa. He first discussed preconceptions and myths about Africa, such as that it is homogeneous; Africa is physically, culturally, and socially very diverse. He then described the lack of health professionals, schools, and demographic data and mentioned communication and transportation problems, linguistic diversity, ethnocentricity, and definitional problems, including debates over certain concepts such as the universality of certain symptoms.

Models developed in Europe and North America for management and control of mental disorder have been transported without much change to local settings in Africa, creating various problems. For example, German (1987) cited the overallocation of health resources to establishing medical schools and technologically advanced hospitals and training of medical specialists; meanwhile, there has been a lack of wide-ranging general practitioner services. Without such a buffer, specialists in mental health are faced with an impossible task and have difficulties functioning in the role for which they have been trained.

German (1987) stated that health services should instead be based on village health workers and other primary health care workers and on development work directed at redressing social evils through education and other means. Social problems must be solved, or mitigated, before sophisticated health techniques can be deployed in any useful way; such problems include alcoholism, drug abuse, breakup of traditional family structures, population mobility due to political upheaval, and socioeconomic shifts. In areas with scarce psychiatric staffing, methods of health care must be rethought to take account of local demographics, socioeconomic conditions, and cultural values.

3

Case 2: The Outraged Nurse

The psychiatrist whose responsibilities include remote rural villages must often also deal with the regional general hospital and other facilities that provide backup services to the villages. The case presented in this chapter illustrates some of the problems that can arise and potential approaches to their understanding and management.

A psychiatrist acting as consultant to a small regional general hospital has responsibility for providing both technical assistance and program monitoring to improve the quality of care in the facility. It might seem that these two roles are rather different, but because of staffing shortages, the consultant must "wear two hats." If his monitoring reveals a problem in a program, he is then supposed to give technical help to fix it. Because the hospital is in a small town 3 hours by plane from the psychiatrist's urban location, site visits to this program are possible only every 3–6 months.

The following letter was sent to the consultant by a nurse in the rural hospital.

June 12, 1987

Dear Dr. X.:

Please find enclosed a copy of a letter I wrote to our local mental health program director. It is self-explanatory of our situation in providing holistic care for our region.

Please let us know what suggestions you have to improve this very serious situation, which concerns us all.

Sincerely,

Acting Director of Nursing

A copy of the following letter was enclosed:

May 17, 1987

Dear Mr. Y.:
  There is agreement in this community that it is imperative and necessary for our hospital to be involved in crises that occur. Certain crises such as suicide attempts mandate hospital staff intervention. However, this service requires the nurse and the physician to be familiar with modern concepts of community mental health, as well as principles of community action.
  To respond competently and efficiently, certain plans and guidelines need to be assessed, evaluated, and implemented.
  In the recent admission of a patient who had attempted suicide, I realized how deficient and ill-equipped we are to assume accountability for treatment we cannot provide without some serious professional consultations and collaboration to improve our program of care.
  To use this particular patient as an example, I must point out the hazards noted. A very suicidal patient was admitted. She then proceeded to slash her wrists right here in our facility. This is outrageous! The physician ordered the patient to be placed on suicidal precaution after she had deeply lacerated both wrists. This order is merely an order to relieve the physician of further accountability. Due to inadequate staffing, the patient was admitted and observed as any regular admission. Aside from this danger, the admission room was unsafe for this particular patient; it contained numerous features that the patient could have used to carry out the original intent . . . suicide. There was an electrical outlet just above the bed. Other dangerous objects, such as the electrical cords for the bed and the call light, the mirror above the sink, plastic liners in the wastepaper basket, and the fact that the door to the bathroom can be locked from the inside, are all important factors to be considered. I'm merely mentioning these few things wrong with the room—there are many more—to emphasize the need for an adequate, safe, receiving room. We need staffing—plus a system to handle these types of dangerous patients—plus a safe room to put them in. This case is just the most recent one; information on several others that were also handled very poorly is attached. Learning what mistakes were made in the past in other institutions can prevent repetition of them at our facility. I have

*been involved in situations elsewhere where patients committed sui-
cide in the hospital and don't want to see us making the very same
mistakes and having needless deaths here!*

*As for accountability, quality assurance requires that the hospi-
tal define its purpose and operationalize its goals so the program and
personnel's performance can be measured against stated objectives.
Documentation is required to demonstrate that changes are made according to what is found. Staff here seem to just be going through the
motions as far as quality assurance.*

*I would greatly appreciate your views in this important matter,
which concerns us all.*

Sincerely,

Acting Director of Nursing

Multiple courtesy copies of this letter were routed to the acting hospital
director, the chief of the regional health department, the newly arrived
medical director of the hospital, and others. (Because of recruiting and
retention problems, there are a number of "actings" and recent arrivals
on the local staff.)

The patient chart information on the woman who slashed her
wrists revealed the following:

1. The patient was 30 years old.
2. She had health records not only in this facility, but in another rural
    health facility, as well as two urban facilities and a rural health
    clinic. However, these records were not immediately available to
    staff who needed them.
3. At the hospital where the nurse worked, the patient had a record
    of visits starting when she was 24 years old. "Chief problems" listed
    on the "active problems" summary included:

April 1984—ingestion of amitriptyline
May 1984—iron overdose; alcohol overdose
January 1986—ingestion of amitriptyline
February 1986—intentional suicide gesture, recurrent (iron over-
dose); intentional alcohol intoxication, chronic
July 1986—head injury
July 1986—contusion, possible strain of left chest wall
August 1986—depression; drug ingestion, unspecified
February 1987—blunt facial trauma
March 1987—ingestion of power-steering fluid

There were other visits on several occasions for urinary tract infections, vaginitis, and family planning.

The page from the chart dealing with the current admission had only a very brief, handwritten note by the admitting doctor. It reported that there had been an ambulance call; the patient had been found unconscious on the bathroom floor, drunk and with a moderate amount of bleeding from self-inflicted lacerations of both wrists from a small knife. She was awakened and was combative and uncooperative. A description of the lacerations and the suturing used was given. The patient had then been admitted. There was no note as to mental status, no suicidal precautions or other treatment plan (that part of the admitting form was left blank), and no consultation requests for the substance abuse or mental health program staff to see her. Although it was not documented in what the nurse sent, it appeared that the patient had made another attempt to slash her wrists after being admitted.

Information on other patients was also included. One had been admitted to the hospital after an overdose but was not put on suicide precautions. He walked up to the nursing station and said he needed a razor to shave. The nursing aide gave him the razor. He went back into his room, but came out a few minutes later with a blood-stained towel wrapped around his neck, which was cut. He was sewn up, then sent back to the same room, again unattended because of staff shortages. He returned a few minutes later, having kicked in the toilet bowl in the room and used a piece of broken porcelain to try to cut himself.

Another patient, admitted after a suicide attempt, had apparently simply walked out of the hospital shortly after admission; it was not clear what the follow-up had been.

This hospital has had severe recruiting and retention problems and extremely high staff turnover. Some of the staff are on temporary duty or locum tenens assignments, and a number of positions are unfilled.

The regional mental health program, located in the same small town but separate from the hospital, is headed by a master's-level psychologist. No psychiatrists or Ph.D. psychologists or psychiatric nurses are available in the region. The former hospital social worker has left, and it has not been possible to fill the position because of funding problems and a scarcity of housing; the staff quarters formerly occupied by the social worker are now filled by a staff physician and his family.

There are no local mental health facilities, and it is difficult to identify the program that the regional mental health program director is supposedly directing. He has been having medical problems lately and has appeared to other staff to be burned out. He has an assistant— a social worker who is looking around for some other job—plus a secretary.

Paraprofessionals who have suicidal patients in the surrounding villages call up the general hospital to speak to a family physician. If the situation seems serious, the patient is flown into town for further evaluations. If there is a medical overlay (e.g., gunshot wound needing surgery, severely slashed wrist, serious overdose) and the patient is voluntary, he or she is admitted to the hospital. The mental health program director or the social worker is then called in for a consult.

Involuntary patients, or serious suicidal patients without a medical overlay, are handled differently. A local magistrate issues a pickup order after a hearing, and a state trooper flies to the village and brings the patient into town to be detained at the regional jail. Then the patient is flown to the nearest psychiatric evaluation facility, which in this case is in the urban center. When weather is too bad for flying, as frequently happens, the patient may spend several days in the jail. (This is another problem; some patients have attempted suicide while in the jail, and the staff there would like some training on what to do, if the psychiatrist can find time on one of his site visits.) The local alcohol program has its own short-term residential treatment facility, but it is staffed by paraprofessionals who feel uncomfortable with substance abusers who are also suicidal or who might have "mental" disorders. Because so many people have substance abuse problems in this community, the facility usually does not have empty beds anyway.

Analyzing a Hospital System

This case occurred in a different rural setting from Case 1, but the dynamic pattern described in Dog Bone's case, of looking for outside help (in this case from the urban psychiatrist/consultant) to fix a local problem is apparent here as well. Similar questions—which level to work at, how much to try to get done at the local level, and whether and when to accede to the request for a "hired gun" or higher authority from outside—must be answered.

Other possible issues present themselves when the hospital is considered as a system. Figure 3–1 gives a schematic view of a hospital system's key processes or flows. Something comes into the system, is processed, and then leaves. In the case of a hospital system, patients are admitted, are assessed and treated, and then are discharged. Both clinical and management staff are recruited, enter the system and work there, and eventually leave for other jobs. There is a facility that the people work in, including equipment and supplies.

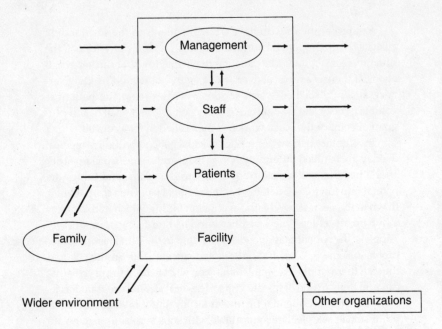

Figure 3–1.   Analysis of a health organization.

Representing the hospital functions in this general way provides a useful conceptual map of where to begin looking for possible problems and intervention points. Using such a map is similar to a radiologist's examining a chest X ray, systematically scanning different areas so as not to miss significant changes.

Elaboration on the basic diagram can be done to depict key functions and departments in more detail. For example, the management functions could be split into those done by various departments (e.g., personnel, finance, planning). The patient intake process could be further elaborated to address outreach, initial contact, triage, and diagnostic assessments. Follow-up and aftercare activities could also be flowcharted in more detail. The basic method involves mapping the processes and then taking a careful look at each subsection to see what improvements might be possible to solve the problem at hand.

The psychiatrist who wants to be maximally helpful in situations involving small, remote facilities cannot look only at individual patients, or at patient-nurse interactions, although these may need to be addressed. Instead, he or she must examine all aspects of the hospital system—how staff are recruited and oriented; staff credentialing and privileging; how management gets feedback from staff and patients; budgetary constraints; and even the facility's architecture and room layout, equipment, and supplies. Any of these may contain potential problems.

This process is similar to a program review done by the Joint Commission on Accreditation of Healthcare Organizations (JCAHO), in which a team looks at all the various aspects affecting quality of care. Here, because of lack of resources for a full team, the psychiatrist does something similar, but with a simplified and less formal schematic in mind. The aim is to determine, quickly but systematically, which key functions to concentrate on to get the most leverage from a brief intervention.

For example, would the best response to the acting director of nursing in Case 2 be to try to shore up the hospital's management so it can set appropriate policies for dealing with suicidal patients? Would it pay off better to try to intervene at the staff level, providing in-service training, or to set up different recruiting, orientation, and retention strategies to improve the chances of finding and keeping top-quality staff? Or would it be best to try to find another facility to take the suicidal patients so they would not get into this hospital system in the first place?

Many other options will emerge as the system is analyzed in terms of what happens first, what next, what follows that, and then each step is critically examined to see what might be modified or improved. The psychiatrist, as well as the other people involved, usually has severely limited resources available to solve problems; after analysis, if a problem can be solved more than one way, the solution that costs least in time and/or money can be chosen. Because a whole array of problems tends to be "unbundled" for presentation to visiting experts, this kind of analysis permits consultants to pick the starting point where the most leverage can be obtained, multiplying the impact of a brief intervention and possibly solving more than one problem at once.

This is very basic systems engineering. It is also similar to core methodology used in "continuous quality improvement," "total quality management," the "Deming method," and a variety of other similar approaches (Scherkenbach 1986). In remote rural and developing areas, a simplified version of these methods can be useful in coming up with a practical problem-solving strategy.

To make the most of this approach, psychiatrists must extend their interests and skills beyond those of a clinician and learn how other elements of the overall system (e.g., the budget officer, the personnel director, the hospital administrator, the facility planner, other clinicians) think about and perform their jobs. Because problems tend to be repeated with minor variations in each small rural facility, it does not take long to acquire expertise in identifying areas that will be easiest to improve and will give maximum results for the time and money involved.

In this case, analysis of the system is a first step to considering such questions as what should happen before patients like this enter the hospital, what should be done at the time of admission, how the patient should be handled while in the hospital, and what kinds of aftercare and follow-up are needed when the patient returns to the remote village. How to involve the patient's family, as well as the larger community and other organizations, in an effective system of care should also be planned and negotiated.

Staffing Problems

Staffing is a serious problem at this hospital. There is an acting rather than full-time hospital director, an acting director of nursing, and temporary or newly arrived staff who have not been oriented well; lack of staff prevents one-to-one supervision of a suicidal patient, and people who ought to be working closely together do not seem to be doing so. Some staff may be burned out or in jobs that are too difficult for them. Who will be working on how staff are recruited and selected, what sort of orientation and in-service training they will get, what incentives can be offered for remaining on the job rather than leaving after short stays, and how can burnout be prevented are just some of the questions that must be considered.

Management Problems

The top management at this facility also seems to be ineffective. The "organizational culture" is not promoting quality. Values and organizational goals are unclear, and budgeting and personnel functions are inadequate. The physical facility is unacceptable; the room used to hold suicidal patients is too far from the nurse's station to permit watching such patients closely, and various dangerous items (e.g., glass windows, metal pipes to hang oneself from, objects that can be easily broken) are in the room. Because renovation costs may be high, however, alternatives to keeping suicidal patients in this hospital at all should be examined, as well as low-cost changes that would increase the patients' safety to the degree possible.

As in the previous case, the psychiatrist makes brief visits to the regional hub town where the general hospital is located only every 3–6 months. Careful thought should be given to how to get the most done in the limited on-site psychiatric time available.

Looking at the Larger Picture

Like Dog Bone, the suicidal patient in this case, far from being an isolated "horror story," is prototypical of a variety of situations in remote rural areas, where suicidal behavior—often alcohol related—is not uncommon. Rural facilities of all kinds are often understaffed or their staff are not well trained in assessing lethality. There is generally high staff turnover, and local management capacity may be very limited. Alcohol is often surprisingly available, even inside facilities. Consultants may therefore get requests for help from rural jails, for example, whose personnel feel they do not know how or do not have enough staff to prevent prisoners from drinking or attempting suicide. Suicide attempts, and sometimes completed suicides, occur in rural alcohol and mental health facilities, as well as in the local jails. In small villages, there may not be a jail or a local alcohol treatment or mental health facility. In these situations, working out a safe place to watch a severely suicidal patient can be a major challenge, especially if weather conditions prevent flying the patient to a regional or urban center.

Who "Owns" the Problem?

In this case, the regional general hospital, whose acting director of nursing wrote to ask for help, is part of the same organization for which the psychiatrist in the urban center works. The hospital, however, is managed autonomously; recruitment, hiring decisions, and staff orientation are carried out as management sees fit. The regional mental health program, on the other hand, gets its funding from another agency and is in a separate building a few blocks away from the hospital. It is thus able to act quite independently from the regional hospital and from the urban psychiatrist. It has different standards, a different data system, and a different set of organizations to which it must respond to comply with requirements of its funding source.

Some of the funding for the programs described in this case comes from the federal government, some from the state, and some from local sources. This is not unusual in rural areas like Alaska, where there is a patchwork of federal, state, and local health organizations, with overlapping and sometimes conflicting organizational responsibilities.

A "memo of agreement" is required between the mental health program and the hospital. However, because of staff turnover at both facilities and the tendency of local clinical staff to view memos of agreement as "administrative b.s." that should be someone else's job, the memo of agreement has not been updated in some time.

Accrediting organizations such as the JCAHO do come to review the general hospital. However, because there are no inpatient psychiatric beds at the hospital, review of the mental health services, which are largely ambulatory, is minimal. Officials from the agency that funds the mental health program feel that more quality assurance of the hospital's mental health services is needed, but because these officials are nonmedical and not familiar with hospital clinical services, they are not aware of how serious the problems are and are not certain how those problems they do know about should be fixed.

As in other cases, it might be argued that the village the patient originally came from, or the patient's family, or the patient herself owns the problem. Certainly, efforts at the village level to reduce the number of suicidal patient admissions to the general hospital should be considered. But the situation within the hospital clearly requires changes.

Many factors contribute to the hospital staff's reluctance to own this patient and her problems. Perhaps most critical is the extreme difficulty the hospital has had in recruiting and retaining staff; closing it down entirely has been actively discussed several times, and only the high cost of flying patients to the urban center has rescued it. The hospital has about 16 beds, with 6 doctors and 12 nurses when fully staffed, plus an administrator and an administrative assistant; this is not much "bench strength" to take up the slack when an experienced staff member leaves. In addition, many staff members came to Alaska to do general medical work, and they resent working in a hospital filled with psychiatric patients.

Thus, a number of people potentially own this situation, but in practice no one does. Patients like this would be difficult to manage well, even if there were clear ownership; chronic personality problems and substance abuse generally contribute to their repeated "parasuicidal" behavior.

State commitment laws allow involuntary commitment of people who make very serious suicide attempts when there is "imminent danger" and a mental disorder. However, the term *mental disorder* is interpreted as requiring a diagnosable condition under Axis I of DSM-IV (American Psychiatric Association 1994). It is therefore difficult to get patients committed when chronic personality problems and substance abuse are predominant. These Axis II disorders are not considered by the psychiatrists at the state commitment facility to meet the definition of mental disorder intended by the commitment law.

Particularly for patients from remote rural areas, it is difficult to get the types of workups done that would document the need for commitment in a way that is convincing to urban staff—often unfamiliar with rural needs—on the receiving end of the commitment. The suicidal patient, like the assaultive patient in Case 1, may seem to be a problem to local people, but not to professionals in distant cities who make the commitment decisions.

The psychiatrist or other mental health professional in these situations is often told immediately by the locals that he or she owns the problem and should fix it right away. This "shifting the burden" dynamic pattern is discussed in Case 1. The role of heroic rescuer and problem solver can be a seductive one; the psychiatrist must try to keep a balance, not getting drawn into unrealistic rescue efforts, but also not backpedaling unduly. Effective solutions are likely to involve many people participating in a problem-solving team; the psychiatrist can often help by keeping track of who will be responsible for what.

What Can Be Done for the Immediate Problem?

Various practical solutions come immediately to mind in this case (e.g., improving at least one holding room in the hospital so it will be safe for suicidal patients, getting policies and procedures in place to deal with restraints, setting up a one-to-one surveillance system, in-service training for staff in lethality assessment and brief treatment). The problem for the local participants and for the urban psychiatrist, however, is what to cut to pay for these new activities; there is not enough funding to hire new staff, do facility renovations, and so on, without cutting back elsewhere. Existing medical and nursing staff, moreover, are uncomfortable at the prospect of dealing with mental patients and are especially leery about involuntary patients, whom their hospital is not set up to handle. They are reluctant to cut acute-care medical activities, which they understand and feel comfortable with, to deal with psychiatric patients.

On the other hand, the psychologist or director of the mental health program feels unprepared to deal with hospital policies and procedures and with training needs of doctors and nurses. (In rural areas, program directors may be people who would not qualify for jobs of similar responsibility in an urban center. Because the local mental health program may be a one- or two-person operation, backing up a nonclinical program manager by hiring a clinical director may not be feasible.)

The psychiatrist can invite the local players to sit down together and discuss how suicide attempters will be handled at each step along the way (e.g., case finding, initial workup, procedures while in the hospital, discharge planning). Because of the high staff turnover, one such meeting is not likely to be enough. Some sort of ongoing teamwork, accommodating a frequently changing cast of characters, will probably need to be developed. The psychiatric consultant should investigate possible ways to accomplish this.

Use of videos about managing the suicidal patient, which could be required as part of new employees' orientation, might be an efficient training method for frequently changing staff. A group of local people could be encouraged to form a quality assurance committee; the committee could use "psychological autopsy" methods to try to identify possible intervention strategies for high-risk patients, including those who make multiple suicide attempts. A variety of other possibilities could be considered, such as convincing local program managers that joint funding of certain positions would allow them to serve a linchpin role.

Reorganizing the System

In this particular case, after consideration of a number of options, it was decided that a key intervention would be filling the vacant social worker position at the hospital. Then there would be someone on staff to work on behavioral health problems full-time. The problems described here were just the tip of the iceberg, so a full-time staff member was clearly needed.

The psychiatrist asked a social worker in the urban center to help write a new job description, to help with the advertising and recruiting, to help orient the new social worker once recruited, and then to provide technical backup by phone. The psychiatrist would provide some specialized in-service training for the new social worker on handling suicidal patients, would assist with quality assurance activities, and periodically would hold a special clinic to assess suicidal patients with the local staff.

This strategy ran into problems; it turned out the hospital had used the funding originally allocated to the social worker position for other purposes during a financial crisis, and the housing formerly reserved for the hospital social worker had been given to another staff member. Because of the shortage of housing in this small town and the expense of living off the hospital compound, it would have been extremely difficult to recruit someone without hospital housing.

Meanwhile, a number of additional technical assistance visits were made by the psychiatrist, along with a team consisting of a social worker, a psychologist, and a substance abuse program specialist, to try to solve the problems raised by the Outraged Nurse. She left before the problems could be solved, and the considerable staff turnover meant that each time the consultants came back, they met a different group of local participants. Extensive teleconferences were held to try to keep costs down.

Eventually, an alternate funding source was found in another agency, which provided enough money to expand the services and to hire another social worker at the regional community mental health center. Then an arrangement was worked out whereby that social worker came to the hospital and worked with the local family physicians to provide additional care for some of the psychiatric patients. Thus, the hospital facility was used, but staff were detailed by another agency to do what otherwise would have been done by a hospital social worker.

Once this base was established, the psychiatrist could restructure his role in a more efficient way. Specialty clinics became possible every 3 months, after the psychiatrist spent time with the central budget officer and found a small amount of additional travel funds in the budget for technical assistance; a billing system developed with the local people may make additional visits possible. During the clinics, the psychiatrist, along with the social worker, made assessments and developed treatment plans for difficult patients. In-service education sessions for local family physicians and other hospital and community-based staff were also held. Between the psychiatrist's visits, the social worker followed up on the treatment plans, telephoning the psychiatrist or consulting with local family physicians as needed.

Subsequently, the program experienced various ups and downs, including crises when the regional mental health program lost funding due to statewide cutbacks and had to lay off staff, burnout of staff, hiring of some staff who were not qualified to do the job, and various management problems. Thus, the psychiatrist was not able to perform a quick fix and solve a problem permanently in a short time. What this case illustrates is the nature of a problem-solving process and the twists and turns the psychiatrist must make over time, being extremely creative and flexible and taking on many nonclinical roles to try to be of practical help.

It is encouraging to note that the problems in this region are slowly improving. In the 1970s, there was no regional mental health program in place at all, and no women's shelter, home for senior citizens, or alcohol treatment facility, all of which are now in place. The villagers do not attach as much stigma to psychiatric patients as in the past and at times are even demanding that more psychiatric services be made available. For the psychiatrist, a long-term perspective leads to understanding that in remote rural settings, significant developments and changes occur slowly over many years.

What Else Could Be Done?

In Alaska, a wide variety of efforts are going on at the village, regional, and statewide levels to deal with and to prevent suicidal behavior. At the village level, where opportunities are very restricted, many people feel trapped. Local jobs are scarce, but most village schools do not prepare villagers very well to go away for advanced training or to compete effectively in big-city job markets.

Several projects are under way to encourage villages to develop cottage industries; others bring village entrepreneurs into local high schools to teach teenagers how to develop business plans that might create meaningful work opportunities in the village. Other programs in the school system involve "peer counselors" or "natural helpers" who assist in early detection and counseling of potential suicide attempters. In some places, Native elders work in special "culture camps" or "Spirit Camps" to teach young people survival skills and cultural values (Craig 1988; McNabb 1991).

Another approach is to develop alternative schools built around Native learning styles, which stress observation; hands-on experience; apprenticeships with elder role models; and use of ceremonies, myths, and other traditional activities. Many Alaska Natives believe that the non-Native educational system has a negative effect on Native youth. In their view, the insistence on non-Native learning methods, emphasizing individual learning and using written materials, is the reason that many students drop out of school, with low self-esteem and experiences of failure.

These Native educators examine the schools as systems, in the same way the hospital is considered as a system in this chapter. They look at every aspect of the schooling: who designs the curriculum (outside experts or a committee of parents and students), how the grading is done (a non-Native method of *A*s through *F*s, with rewards for individual excellence and stigmatization of failure, or a Native style rewarding completion of group tasks and de-emphasizing failure), how the students are motivated (using non-Native school counselors or traditional role models, talking circles, and other forms of Native group therapy), and so on. Problems such as suicidal behavior will be much less likely to develop if the local culture considers school dropouts and other problem teenagers not as failures with learning disabilities and other pathology, but as people with alternative learning styles who need to be encouraged and strengthened through traditional Native methods before they become suicidal.

Other efforts to prevent suicidal behavior include programs on parenting, village health fairs where suicide is discussed among other topics, health education classes, poster contests, and community minigrants aimed at developing local innovative approaches. Village response teams get special training in how to respond to emergencies, including suicide attempts. Some communities see the problem as partly one of culture breakdown, in which outsiders' efforts to "civilize" and modernize Native life resulted in breakdown of traditional cultural and social supports and increased problems such as alcoholism and suicide. In a number of communities, this line of thinking is leading to reestablishing traditional cultural ceremonies.

Regional Projects

At the regional level, suicide-attempter registries are being set up with systematic protocols; these allow improved follow-up of patients. For example, in one region a registry was kept for 4 years of all suicide attempts and completed suicides. In this time period, there were 200 total incidents—176 attempts and 24 completed suicides. This is almost one attempt per week, and about one completed suicide every 2 months, in a total population of 7,000. The computerized registry contains basic data about the persons involved, such as identifying information, the nature of the suicide attempt, available information on health status, past history of suicide attempts, and family history.

Working with these data, the psychiatrist and social workers in the region are carrying out simple analyses. For example, about 70 of the 200 incidents occurred in people under age 20; 22 of those were in people ages 15 or younger. Because this group, which is starting early with suicidal behavior, appears to be at high risk for future attempts or completions, it is being singled out for special study. The consulting psychiatrist will try to determine what has happened over the past 4 years to these young attempters, using information in the general hospital medical charts and other agency information, vital statistics data, and information from local health providers. For those who have completed suicides relatively recently, psychological autopsies can be carried out. The analysis can be presented to local tribal health authorities, with the goal of mobilizing them to write grant proposals for prevention, treatment, and follow-up programs.

This project exemplifies one type of population-based activity with which psychiatrists may be involved. Their clinical skills are used in reviewing the histories of the attempters, looking for risk indicators and early warning signs, developing intervention strategies, and setting up special suicide clinics. They also use various nonclinical skills, however, such as presenting to tribal authorities, writing grant proposals, organizing programs, training paraprofessionals, evaluating programs, and finding people with such skills to be part of a team.

Other activities may include getting local providers to sit down together and work out protocols—for example, deciding in advance who will do the medical screening for the suicidal emergency patient, where the severely suicidal patient will be admitted, what will happen if the patient is "dual diagnosis," how cases that must be referred out-of-region will be handled, how "high users" of the system will be handled, and what will be done for an involuntary patient or a minor. On-call systems need to be set up, and decisions must be made about what to cut unless new monies or staff time are available. Building of special programming for young suicide attempters is still at a beginning stage; Case 3 in Chapter 4 involves an example of programming that is further along.

Religious organizations, both at the village and the regional levels, may also need to be involved. Fundamentalist groups, common in rural Alaska, may be opposed to efforts to encourage Native "Spirit Programs." On the other hand, they may be helpful in providing support groups for certain patients and family members, along with some degree of aftercare and follow-up.

Efforts at the State Level

At the statewide level, advocacy for programs for suicidal patients; encouragement of funding for research and training efforts; and demonstration "suicide clinics" to show how teams can evaluate, treat, and follow up on suicidal patients are useful efforts by individuals or groups. Program review systems can be set up to focus on problems, such as those described in this case, that are being missed by JCAHO or other program monitoring.

What Should the Psychiatrist's Role Be?

Like Dog Bone's case in Chapter 2, this case shows how important it is for clinicians in remote rural areas to be able to take on new roles—as policymakers, planners, advocates, backup for midlevel practitioners, trainers and coaches for paraprofessionals, and so on. They may need to assist local managers, such as the acting hospital director and the Outraged Nurse in this case, as well as clinicians and patients, to have maximum impact. This means that role definition by the psychiatrist is essential. Otherwise, the role will be defined by the local people, who often tend to do "business as usual," involving the psychiatrist mainly as a technician to do medical checks or else making unrealistic demands that the psychiatrist solve the problem single-handedly.

Goal Erosion

One way to conceptualize this case is to look at how pressures associated with the remote rural location have created "goal erosion" (Senge 1990b). Some local staff are aware of what should be done for suicidal patients, but staffing and facility problems seem almost insurmountable. Under these conditions, people often start to adjust their sights so that the original goals of providing high-quality health care are progressively lowered. The pressure to lower goals leads to further reduction in expectations.

New people coming into a situation where goal erosion has occurred cannot get a clear idea of what the organization should be doing. Soon everyone is heading off in different directions in a fragmented way.

Reversing Goal Erosion

To reverse this process, the psychiatrist can exert leadership both directly and indirectly to clarify or revivify goals. To do this, the psychiatrist must have the goals clearly in mind and must be able to communicate them effectively to others.

Since the psychiatrist is not on the scene, local leaders and team builders must be found; the psychiatrist will have to identify these people and decide how best to support them. The local leaders should be people who can get everyone aimed in the same direction, with a strong sense of purpose and clear goals—processes called "goal alignment" and "building shared vision" (Senge 1990b). Usually this means they are strong personal examples of what they believe in and are adept at using words, comfortable and effective in addressing others, able to work well in groups, "other-centered" rather than self-ambitious, mature in human relationships, persistent, and innovative. If such people are available and can be encouraged, the psychiatric consultant's job becomes much easier.

Example From Another Setting

The following example demonstrates one of the tasks involved in this case: that of standing outside the clinical role, "de-centering" from it (to use an anthropological term), and looking at a health care system and one's own role from an outsider's point of view. This process can help identify overall system problems.

Presenting to an Attending

In this example, medical anthropologists are studying a hospital system (Muller 1993). They are particularly interested in how interactions between doctors and patients are perceived, interpreted, and given meaning within a clinical context. This is similar to what rural psychiatrists must do, looking at interactions, normally taken for granted, in terms of the various participants' goals and possible problematic aspects. What happens in this example is not unlike what may happen in busy small general hospitals with the local family physicians.

The anthropologists decide to study medical students presenting recently worked-up cases to an attending senior physician. Each student must demonstrate a process of constructing the patient's story and retelling it in an accepted format. Anthropologists consider this a form of ritual. The consultant interprets the story, identifying salient information and missing data. The student is evaluated on how well the data are gathered, organized, and presented.

The hospital system is a large, complex inner-city system, with multiple forms to be filled out on each patient, ever-present time pressures, and translation problems with the culturally diverse patient population. The students are expected to function as primary physicians, but they get less supervision and more responsibility than they might in other settings. Because patient visits with the students often take longer than expected, patients and charts back up. The training program stresses family history, psychosocial history, and continuity of care, but how much information is collected depends on how much time is available.

The students are observed by the anthropologists as they make their presentations to the attendings and also in their work with the patients. Interview information from the participants is also collected.

The students want to make a good impression; to show they are clinically competent, thorough, and responsible; and to reassure the attending that they can be trusted so that they will get good evaluations for the rotation. There is considerable pressure to make a plan and get finished, instead of opening a Pandora's box of psychosocial problems.

The students therefore emphasize some information and de-emphasize other data if they did not get it or were pressed for time. The students also set boundaries for what they feel responsible for knowing. This extends even to the point of tuning out attendings who give them information that seems too abstract and not what they think they need for that patient.

What sort of socialization process is taking place with these trainees? What will be their sensitivity to psychological and social issues such as those that occur in a remote rural hospital setting once they have completed this type of training?

4

Case 3: Pregnant but Dead

Case 3 illustrates the "systems building" activities that psychiatrists and other participants in multidisciplinary efforts undertake in the process of creating new programs that will fill gaps in existing rural services. Like some of the other cases, the problem presents initially as an individual patient. Because there are a large number of people with similar problems, however, the psychiatrist's clinical work needs to be supplemented with a population-based approach.

A 29-year-old woman hanged herself and died. She was 6 months pregnant at the time of death, and the fetus did not survive. The psychiatrist is asked to review her medical records to determine whether anything can be done to prevent future deaths like this. There are two charts, each several inches thick. The patient had one chart at the rural hospital in the small town where she grew up. The second chart is at an urban hospital where she made frequent visits in the past year since moving into the city. These are both general medical hospitals. It is difficult to piece together a complete story from the charts. Most of the notes are very brief, some made in the emergency room, mainly describing the physical findings with little social history or psychological information. The psychiatrist is able to reconstruct the following.

The patient spent most of her life in the small town where she was born. Virtually nothing is recorded in the charts about her family background or early development. Starting at about age 13, she began a pattern of abusive drinking. Visits were noted every 2–3 months to the rural hospital's emergency room for minor injuries, intoxication, and venereal diseases.

Beginning at age 15, the patient was pregnant a total of six times, with two abortions. She was reported to be drinking about a fifth of vodka per day throughout her first pregnancy, which went to term. The baby was small for its age, with features suggestive of fetal alcohol effects but not the full-blown fetal alcohol syndrome. She took the baby home, but after 3 months the court decided she was an unfit parent because of her heavy drinking, and she lost custody of her child. Her boyfriend also reportedly was a heavy drinker, and several of her emergency room visits were for injuries reportedly caused by her boyfriend's abuse.

Heavy drinking continued during the later pregnancies. Both babies had fetal alcohol syndrome. One had severe heart problems, sometimes associated with fetal alcohol syndrome, and died at 5 months. The other was removed from the home shortly after delivery because the patient was found passed out on the street from intoxication on several occasions.

During these years, attempts were made to involve her in programs offered by the local alcohol project. However, she was highly resistant, denied she had problems, and screamed at the emergency room staff when this was suggested, then stormed out. The local alcohol program meanwhile had multiple reorganizations and staff turnover. It was not set up to provide in-depth evaluation or counseling, but mainly provided sleep-off, followed by referrals to Alcoholics Anonymous. No residential treatment was available locally. There was a social worker at the hospital, but no mental health or psychiatric services. The rural hospital was extremely small—only 12 beds—with a staff of four physicians who seldom stayed more than a year or two, a small nursing staff, and a small support staff.

When her third baby was taken away, the patient was very angry. She showed up drunk on numerous occasions at the children's group home and at various foster homes where the child was placed, making threats to harm the foster parents if her baby was not returned. Her threats were clearly effective; the child had been in seven different foster placements by the age of 2. The mother was also angry with the welfare workers, and the town's small size meant that she was often in contact with them as well as with the various foster parents.

During the last year of her life, the patient moved to the city, for reasons that were not entirely clear. She must have had considerable problems in adjusting; she had lived all her life in a small town, had apparently dropped out of school at about age 14, and had no job skills. This, however, was not recorded in the chart. She made 25 visits to the city hospital's emergency room in the year prior to her death—a visit about once every 2 weeks. On most of these visits, she stated she was drinking one- to two-fifths of vodka a day. She was picked up and brought to the emergency room several times by the police after passing out on the street.

On three occasions, she said she had been raped. Men had picked her up in bars, then taken her to hotel rooms or apartments and attacked her. On one visit, she had bad burns on her inner thighs from a coffeepot. There was also a bout with hepatitis.

She became pregnant 6 months before her death, but did not come in for prenatal care until the fourth month. She said she wanted to stop drinking, so she wouldn't lose her baby. However, she signed out "against medical advice" 2 days after entering a residential treatment center. She did not keep subsequent prenatal appointments, but she did show up frequently at the emergency room after being picked up for intoxication, injuries, and an episode of epigastric pain with a possible bleeding ulcer. She stayed for a short while at a boarding home, but then went back to her boyfriend, who was also drinking heavily.

There was no mention in the charts of attempts to refer to psychiatry or social services. The notes were very brief—usually a copy of the pickup findings by the community service patrol, a blood alcohol level, and a short comment as to physical status. No notes as to mental status, depression, or suicidal intention were recorded.

She was found by her boyfriend partially supported by a chair in a hotel room, with a sheet wrapped around her neck and attached to a light fixture on the ceiling. She apparently had stood on the chair, then stepped off to hang herself. She remained in a coma for the next month; every effort was made to prolong her life in the hope that the fetus could be saved. However, she died in intensive care with pneumonia and a cardiac arrhythmia, and the fetus did not survive.

After reviewing these charts, the psychiatrist asks how many pregnant women in this area drink during their pregnancies. In the population served by this hospital system, there could be as many as 800 per year. Of these, between 10 and 50 drink as heavily as the patient that died. About two-thirds of this group are in small, rural, isolated communities; the others are in the city.

Developmental Histories of Psychiatric Problems

A whole book could be written about this case. Over the course of this woman's life, numerous people in many different places attempted to help her without success.

A "lifeline" diagram, similar to Table 4–1, can illustrate a problem's

Table 4–1.　Case 3's lifeline: a developmental history

Ages (years)					
0–13 years	13	14	15–28	28–29	29
No information available	Abuse of alcohol; minor injuries; venereal disease	Dropped out of school	6 pregnancies; 2 abortions; lost custody of child; abuse from boyfriend; 2 fetal alcohol syndrome babies	Moved to city; emergency room visits; drinking; rapes; burns; hepatitis; no prenatal care	Suicide

developmental history and can suggest ways from a public health point of view that high-risk people might be targeted at various points in the developmental process. Such lifeline diagrams are especially useful with groups of paraprofessionals and others who will have to work together.

This kind of lifeline diagram can succinctly summarize many "inches" of medical records and increase awareness of longer-term trends that are not so obvious when the focus is on the immediate presenting problem or crisis. Patients (as well as families, villagers, or other types of groups) can chart similar "time lines"; they encourage dynamic and developmental analyses of how problems have arisen and what might be done. There are many variations of the basic time-line diagram. For example, a vertical dimension can be added so that the patient's high points and low points at various times can be graphically displayed.

Keeping in mind the general principle that early intervention is preferable, would any interventions have been possible with this patient before age 13, which was the earliest detection of alcohol abuse, injuries, and venereal disease? What steps might have been taken between age 15 and her untimely demise at age 29? The lifeline diagram suggests a number of possible intervention points, involving schools, prenatal clinics, and emergency rooms, as well as mental health and substance abuse programs, welfare workers, and so on.

Who "Owns" the Problem?

As in the previous cases, a large number of people could be named as "owners" of the problem. The patient's medical records at just one of the hospitals consisted of several volumes 3 inches thick. She had been seen at other hospitals, as well as a number of other institutions.

Here, as in other cases, the psychiatrist could define the problem as "not my job" and wait for a better patient. Or the psychiatrist could get involved as part of a multidisciplinary team, taking ownership of at least portions of the problem and attempting to create programs to deal with it. To avoid the "shifting the burden to the outside intervener" pattern, whatever is done must incorporate considerable community education and involvement. Because the teams working on this kind of problem may involve obstetricians, pediatricians, psychiatrists, nurses, patient educators, substance abuse counselors, and a host of others, goal setting and building a shared vision are important.

What Can Be Done for the Immediate Problem?

Since the patient is now dead, it is too late to do anything for her; the psychiatrist or other mental health professional might carry out a psychological autopsy. The psychiatrist could try to locate the patient's relatives and help them with their grief.

This woman, over a lengthy period, had a whole series of "fixes" that failed. Recycling such patients repeatedly through emergency rooms does little to address their fundamental problems. This patient consumed many hours of acute care but never got the rehabilitation she needed to be able to maintain sobriety, to get an education or job skills, and to take care of herself and her family.

A two-pronged approach that addresses both the immediate situation and the fundamental problems is clearly needed. Realistically, however, it can be extremely difficult to do anything beyond constant quick fixes. Many of the staff working in public programs are doctors doing payback of student loans or younger doctors right out of school. Other staff who may have been with the program for years may be either burned out or deadwood and are often unwilling to change their routines. These staff may be neither motivated nor sufficiently skilled to step back from the quick-fix mentality and consider broader-based solutions. When patients come in and demand immediate help, the easiest solution is to spend 15 minutes with them to "get them off your back." If there is a choice between two patients, one known to be a chronic repeater with behavioral problems like the woman in the case presented in this chapter and the other with a serious medical problem such as a myocardial infarction, few staff members will take more than a quick-fix approach to the first patient. It takes time and energy to say, "Wait a minute! Where are we going? Let's take a few moments and figure out what's wrong with the overall process."

The psychiatrist working in a remote rural setting will find that an either-or approach to the situation does not achieve much positive progress. The quick fixes will need to continue while efforts to improve the underlying situation are encouraged.

What Else Could Be Done?

In rural settings, the psychiatrist, along with many others, often must take on a larger and more complex set of responsibilities than would be expected in an urban setting. For example, in this case, the psychiatrist was asked to help develop a comprehensive new program for a whole class of patients.

A young doctor right out of school may be the first or only psychiatrist in the region and may have to deal with newly emerging problems of enormous scope. It is not unusual to have more than one major problem to deal with simultaneously. In the course of a year or so, the psychiatrist might be asked to develop a new program for fetal alcohol syndrome and also to "please do something for children who are inhalant abusers," or to develop a child advocacy center as well as a system of regional child protection teams. This all comes under the job description category of "other duties as assigned," but regular clinical activities do not go away while the psychiatrist is spending time developing new programs.

It is important, therefore, to become expert at personal time management skills, including conceptualizing end results, team building, and delegation skills, to leverage one's own time and effectiveness as much as possible. Leadership and breadth of vision are called for—skills often not developed as well as they might be in today's world of increasing subspecialization in the technical professional schools.

In this case in Alaska, the psychiatrist worked as part of a team with a number of other people—health educators, pediatricians, obstetricians, infant learning specialists, maternal and child health workers, teachers, and school administrators. A whole program of preventative as well as direct service efforts was built up:

1. Chart reviews and summaries were made of a number of cases similar to the one presented here.
2. The scope of the problem was determined. Infant learning program staff, pediatricians, family practitioners, and others were given checklists developed to screen for high-risk children. Those who appeared to have possible fetal alcohol syndrome and were under age 5 were then seen by a dysmorphologist at specially scheduled rural clinics. The under-5 group was selected because the information on the children would be more recent; older children might more easily be lost to follow-up, and evaluating all children rather than just those under 5 would swamp the system. This attempt to identify all possible suspected cases, with verification of diagnosis by a specialist, would help establish a true incidence rate as a baseline for the population. Annual clinics for those born in subsequent years were also set up to bring new cases into the system and to update information. The children were assessed to determine individual treatment needs and how well these needs were being met by the current service providers.
3. Major public education campaigns were developed to build public awareness of the problem, so there would be political support for additional funding. Television, radio, newspapers, posters, and guest speakers were used to convey information; town meetings, village health fairs, and school programs were held; warning labels were put into use; a Fetal Alcohol Syndrome Awareness Week was established; and nondrinking social events were promoted and encouraged. Targeted public education included special programs, some using puppets or comic books, for children, especially girls, before they reached childbearing age, and alcohol awareness lessons in school starting at age 5 (Figure 4–1).
4. Funding was obtained for full-time fetal alcohol syndrome coordinators to work on the project, both at the statewide level and in regional hub towns.
5. Evaluation and counseling programs for high-risk pregnant women visiting prenatal clinics were developed (Figure 4–2).
6. Registry systems were set up to track mothers and high-risk children after birth.
7. Proposals were written, and eventually funded, to establish a resi-

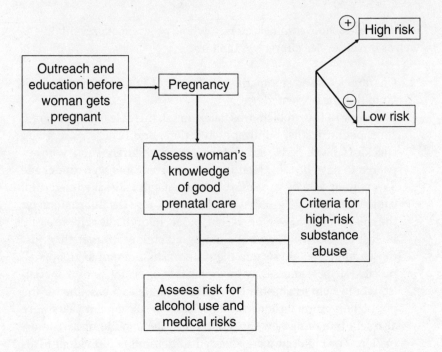

Figure 4–1.   Fetal alcohol syndrome program: assessment of a pregnant mother.

dential treatment program for pregnant substance abusers.

8. Additional links were developed with epidemiologists to allow more tracking and research on the milder cases ("fetal alcohol effect" and "exposed but not currently affected" children).

9. Programs with schools, and with foster parents struggling to take care of difficult children, were eventually established. Training provided for health workers, teachers, and other child care workers included both general material and specific information on screening methods, the referral system, and treatment.

What Should the Psychiatrist's Role Be?

Not everyone will work in a public health setting where the particular problem of fetal alcohol syndrome is prevalent. Nevertheless, the activities sketched indicate the variety of projects with which a remote rural

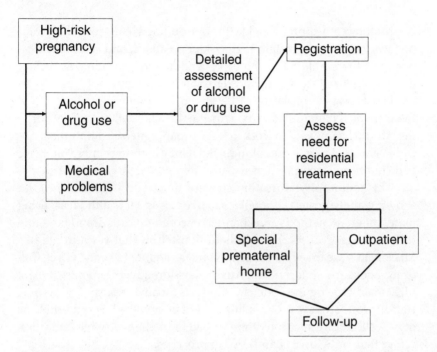

Figure 4–2. Fetal alcohol syndrome program: assessment of a high-risk pregnant mother.

psychiatrist may potentially be involved: 1) assessing difficult patients in prenatal clinics, 2) developing case-finding and community education strategies, 3) developing political support for new funding, 4) planning new facilities, 5) helping with clinical services and in-service professional training, and 6) assisting with psychiatric aspects of research projects. The utmost flexibility and creativity are required, plus an ability to work well with teams, to be a generalist, and to master new parts of projects as they evolve.

In some communities, more than 50% of the residents have severe drinking problems; the norm is to be a drinker, and nondrinkers are considered deviant by most of the community. When problems are so deeply embedded in the social system, individual case approaches may not be very effective. There are usually pennies' worth of resources and many dollars' worth of unmet needs. Standard epidemiological approaches, focusing on describing and analyzing individual cases, also do not work as well with behavioral problems that are entrenched in social and community norms.

Multifaceted approaches like the one outlined here—blending chart reviews, targeting of certain high-risk populations, and case identification, and then building up both prevention and education, as well as direct specialized treatment and rehabilitation programs—appear to be the key. Heavy emphasis must be placed on community change, and there are possibilities, such as convincing the whole village to "vote dry," that would be unlikely to work in large urban centers. Community education is a large part of the solution, but it may have to be more intensive and "multilevel" than what is usually attempted in urban settings.

The community education concept described here goes beyond showing a few posters. It involves marketing social health ideas, using many different methods and channels of communication, and targeting different age groups. The kinds of marketing that restaurants like McDonald's use to sell hamburgers could be adapted to good effect. Coloring books for children, extensive television advertisements, Ronald McDonald-type figures, extensive budgets for advertising, and full-time staff to work on new product lines might be involved. Social problems may well require methods that are likely to change public attitudes, rather than individual "Band-Aid" approaches.

Limited resources in rural areas make targeting necessary. It sometimes appears that a disproportionate amount of time, energy, and money is being spent on a tiny piece of a pervasive problem. Without such targeting, however, the individual psychiatrist is likely to be swamped and to have minimal impact on anything.

5

Case 4: The Long-Haired Psychiatrist

Case 4 illustrates some of the interprofessional problems that can arise in remote rural areas where staff are stretched thin, roles are often unclear, and differences in values can be more problematic than in locations where both professionals and patients have more options (Kates 1993; Keller and Murray 1982; Pathman et al. 1992; Rabinowitz 1993; Will and Baird 1984).

A rural hub town, population 3,000, has the only hospital available for 7,000 people scattered in eight small villages. It is a small general hospital with 15 beds. The geographic area covered is about the size of the state of Montana.

Psychiatric services are limited. There is just one psychiatrist who sees outpatients and consults on the inpatient medical wards. People in the villages fly for 30 minutes to 2 hours to this hub town for many health services; for more specialized care, they may have to fly to the urban center several hours away.

Because there are many more public patients demanding psychiatric services than can be seen by the available staff, the incentive at the rural hospital is to do brief treatment, often with an emphasis on psychotropic medications. The doctors are full-time salaried employees, and there is minimal monitoring of their work; they will keep getting paid even if care is not of high quality. Staff tend to be young psychiatrists right out of school, who work for 1–2 years in public service and then leave, often before learning much about the local culture.

Because airfare to the urban center is expensive, there is next to no choice of providers. The patient's alternatives are to go to the only public program in town or to be a "did not keep appointment" and quit.

An experienced senior psychiatrist works in the urban center in another part of the same general hospital system. As often happens to psychiatrists who stay on in public programs, he has been given more administrative responsibilities and now sees patients only part-time.

A Native woman calls the senior psychiatrist to ask his advice. She had been his patient some years before, after having been raped, and had done extremely well. She tells him, "I'm very concerned about my uncle. He's in his 50s and has spent most of his life in the village. He's been a hard-working fisherman all his life and also flies an airplane. But he doesn't speak English very well and doesn't always feel comfortable expressing himself to white people.

"He's been going over to see the doctors at the hospital in our town for the past 4 months. He had a nervous breakdown. He didn't hear voices or anything like that. I think he was mainly depressed about some close relatives who died in a plane crash.

"He got assigned to see that young psychiatrist—the one with the real long hair who looks like he's a hippie or something. People here in town are always talking about how he doesn't fit in. The doctor put my uncle on Stelazine and some other medicine that starts with an A— I can't remember the name.

"I think there's a real communication problem between my uncle and that doctor. My uncle says he feels uncomfortable with a young doctor anyway, especially somebody with long hair like that. And Uncle's just not like his old self. He seems sort of doped up on the medicine. He's been happily married for 29 years—raised three good kids. He's not crazy or anything like that. Mainly I think he needs someone to talk with about his grief.

"I went with him to see the psychiatrist last time to try to help. I've been to bigger cities some so I feel more comfortable than he does with counselors. But the doctor didn't seem to want to talk much at all. He mainly just read through the chart and then asked if there were any side effects from the medicines. My uncle really felt uncomfortable and couldn't open up at all, even with me there to help. It was a real short visit too.

"I'd like to switch doctors and have my uncle travel in to see you instead. But I don't want to hurt the feelings of the other doctor. And he seemed like he'd be kind of touchy if we asked about changing to a new doctor. Plus someone would need to authorize travel for us—plane tickets are getting real expensive. We do have relatives we could stay with if we can get to the city.

"I don't want to do anything to make problems for you, but I always remember how helpful you were to me in my own case. I'm so grateful. I just want to get my uncle some help, and I know you could really help him. What should I do?"

There is a good possibility that the woman's description of the situation is accurate. The younger doctor has a reputation of doing rather brief workups on patients and sometimes medicating inappropriately. Nevertheless, although he is probably not looking for extra work, the patient's request to switch doctors is likely to offend him.

Because of the small size of the town and limited number of physicians, the patient does not have a choice of psychiatrists if he stays there. He cannot afford the plane fare to see the more experienced psychiatrist recommended by his niece. If the government pays for his ticket, travel authorization forms will have to be approved, and the patient's dissatisfaction with his doctor will come to light. In a small town, there is apt to be a lot of discussion about why this patient is getting special treatment.

On the other hand, it is possible that the niece is distorting the situation. The senior psychiatrist has had some experience with patients and their relatives who wanted special treatment; some people abused the system, wanting their travel paid so they could come to the city for other purposes. In addition, if the patient is really depressed or psychotic, it might not work out well for him to stay with relatives, especially if assessment and treatment take a long time. There could be a real placement problem, because the niece would have to get back home to her job, and local public facilities are all packed.

In this particular case, the patient is older than the doctor and does not speak English very well. He also is not used to talking about personal problems with a younger person. In his own traditions, counselors have to be older than the person being counseled; their greater age and experience make them wiser. Even a very skillful interviewer might well have difficulty communicating with this patient, especially if depression or psychotic features are present.

Who "Owns" the Problem?

Ownership can be unclear because of interprofessional differences and conflicts, which can have multiple causes (Will and Baird 1984). Some stem from psychological factors and personality differences. Certain types of patients, families, and organizations seem to generate interprofessional differences. Other conflicts result from the divergent value systems and perspectives created by different kinds of jobs.

In remote rural areas and in developing countries or regions, programs carried out by the public sector often have unclear and overlapping responsibilities. Thus, a typical clinical or organizational situation involves many people. Various types of "splitting" at several levels—organizational, familial, and individual—occur frequently, and the mental health professional can help by anticipating and preparing to deal with them.

Figure 5–1 displays some of the organizational relationships described in this case. Standard types of organizational charts deal mainly with formal lines of communication. There are also informal patterns of decision making that may differ substantially from what the organizational chart indicates. In remote rural locations, the small numbers of persons interacting in particular situations can lead to fairly serious mismatches between formal and informal communications, and the remote rural psychiatric consultant often must contend with this issue. Diagrams like Figure 5–1 can be useful in clarifying possible ways to resolve organizational communication problems (Kim 1992).

In rural areas, the local public organization often has a parent organization that provides money, standards, technical assistance, monitoring, and so on. More experienced staff tend to gravitate into the parent organization and take on administrative roles. Younger, less experienced staff tend to be on the firing line of the local organization,

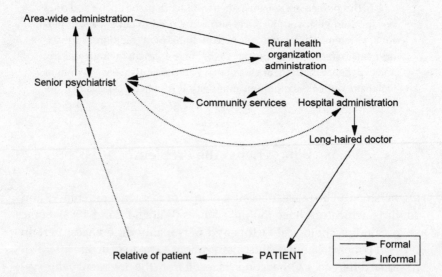

Figure 5–1. Communication lines.

providing direct services and often swamped with large numbers of patients.

Genuine differences in job conditions and definitions can contribute to problems. The consultant can often, within limits, choose which cases to work with, whereas the more generic staff in field units and local departments have restricted ability to select what to take on. Statutory or job design constraints may require them to take certain kinds of difficult patients or a high volume of patients; the consultant usually does not have this same pressure.

Such differences can provide fertile ground for resentment. The consultant may see the local staff as "putting on Band-Aids" or not taking the time or doing the kinds of comprehensive assessments needed for quality work. The local staff, on the other hand, may see the consultant as being in an ivory tower, removed from the reality they have to deal with, or as a paper-pusher or administrative type who does not have to do the frontline work they do. The consultant's relationships with families and community members may also differ greatly from those of the field clinician, often because of the consultant's service on advisory boards or long-term involvement in other community activities and relationships.

The result can be mutual scorn and indignation. The consultant may look down on the work of the local staff and at times feel that his or her specialized experience is being questioned. The local staff may be unappreciative of the consultant's point of view or feel that, even if they would like to take the approach the consultant recommends, their work conditions prevent them from doing so.

Patients often contribute to the problem. When they are not happy with the help they get from the field facility, it is not uncommon for them or their relatives to "buck it upstairs" to someone at a higher level who appears to be responsible. Such a strategy is certainly not unique to rural areas, but it often has a special intensity because rural patients do not have the same range of choice as those in urban settings. If a local provider is the only game in town, switching to another local provider is not possible.

In addition, in rural areas, people may have reasons for wanting to switch doctors that are less common in urban areas. Because small towns tend to be conservative, and to be glass bowls in which very little can be kept secret, personal characteristics of the psychiatrist (e.g., hair length, consumption of alcohol, involvement with a significant other without being married) may be widely known and, indeed, gossiped about all over town. Nonverbal aspects of communication (e.g., degree of eye contact, loudness and tone of voice, firmness of handshake) may also be important to patients. Styles that are valued in one culture, such as a firm handshake, direct eye contact, and questions to find out about problems, may turn off people from another culture who value a softer handshake, less confrontational eye contact, and a noninterference style of observing quietly and waiting until the other person feels comfortable enough to open up about a problem. In addition, remote rural patients may expect more personalized attention; how much time the doctor spends with them and how much effort is made to understand their concerns may be sensitive issues.

Thus, whatever the technical proficiency of the mental health professional, other factors may be of more concern to the patients. A psychiatrist who is sensitive and skilled in one setting may come across as abrasive and insensitive in another. Patients may then try to solve the problem by doing as the niece did in this case: calling on some other professional they know to try to work around their assigned therapist.

Because lines of responsibility both within and between organizations are often vague, problems similar to the one in this case are quite common.

Other Situations Involving Divided Loyalties

The flip side of the problem can occur when a psychiatrist in a rural area is popular. Because so few other mental health professionals are available, the psychiatrist may not ask for help as soon as he or she should. The psychiatrist can get drawn into wearing multiple hats, taking on potentially conflicting roles.

For example, a member of an advisory board that sets policy for the psychiatrist's organization may ask the psychiatrist to provide psychiatric services to a relative or even to the board member. Or a program manager may be referred to a psychiatrist higher up in the same organization, because rural remote areas often lack the independent employee assistance programs that would be available in urban centers.

Some conflicts are between the administrative and the clinical roles, but there are others as well. For example, Congress may require by law that a Federal Indian Health Service psychiatrist "promote Indian self-determination" by monitoring tribal programs and then giving technical assistance when problems are found. It is extremely difficult to do both these jobs well—if monitoring uncovers problems, the psychiatrist has created more work for him- or herself in the technical assistance area. On the other hand, programs may be reluctant to reveal needs for technical assistance, because a negative statement on a program evaluation document could affect future funding. In this instance, two different administrative roles are in conflict: It is hard to be a good-guy technical assistant and a bad-guy inspector at the same time.

Interprofessional tensions can occur if a member of one professional's family needs medical or psychiatric attention. For example, a wife of a psychiatrist in one rural area needed surgery; it was performed by the leading surgeon in the community, but complications developed. The psychiatrist then sought consultation in a nearby city. The original surgeon, one of the leaders of the medical staff at the local hospital, was offended. He began to make unfavorable comments about the psychiatrist's judgment, causing a long period of unpleasantness between the psychiatrist and his colleagues (Jones and Parlour 1985).

Another example might be a staff person whose daughter develops a problem such as cocaine abuse. Extremely concerned, the staff person requests the help of the only psychiatrist in the town. The psychiatrist might like to help, but will have to continue to work closely with the staff person. It may well turn out that the cocaine abuse is associated with numerous conflicts between the daughter and the staff person. On the other hand, if the psychiatrist does not get involved, the staff person will be very unhappy, because other options for treatment locally are almost nonexistent. The staff person may express his or her dissatisfaction to other staff members, complain to the psychiatrist's supervisor, or in other ways put tremendous pressure on the psychiatrist to get involved.

Being the only game in town may result in conflicts that would be much less likely to occur in locations where alternate resources are readily available.

Special Patients and "Splitting"

In addition to scarce resources and organizational problems, psychological dynamics between remote rural patients and urban-trained psychiatrists can lead to problems. Certain patterns tend to appear, particularly those involving "special" patients (Gabbard 1986).

Special patients are often characterized by character pathology resembling that of borderline patients. Primitive defensive operations, such as splitting, projective identification, and denial, are prominent. These patients are frequently self-destructive and suicidal, and this dimension may lead to extraordinary measures to "save" the patient.

Many of these patients have suffered real physical or sexual abuse at the hands of parents and other significant figures. The history of abuse results in patients being seen as victims by everyone because they have, in reality, been victimized; it may also prevent both treaters and patients from seeing the patients' role in perpetuating their own victimization at the hands of others. In addition, this history of victimization is usually accentuated by bad experiences with previous treaters, which make the patients seem even more victimized.

The "victim" role may cause the therapist to overtreat in a zealous attempt to be a loving and devoted parental figure who will make reparation for the damage done to the patient in the past. This attitudinal stance in the treater leads to "overdoing" and to concessions that would not ordinarily be granted. The patient may create feelings of guilt in the treater by suggesting that the patient's own intense negative transference reactions are related to *real* mistreatment and that if only the treatment had been done in a different way, the patient would not have experienced such negative feelings.

Typically, a special patient selects one or two special treaters toward whom an idealized transference develops. The patient then makes these transference objects feel special because they have figured out the right way to treat this patient, almost as though they are psychically attuned to the patient's needs. The other treaters feel they must be doing something wrong because they have not been able to find the mysterious key to eliciting the patient's positive feelings; they frequently give extra attention to such a patient in the hope of discovering how to make the patient respond positively. In contrast, there are other borderline patients who are persistently negative to everyone in the treatment environment; they are often written off as simply obnoxious or unsalvageable, and they do not inspire the devoted therapeutic efforts that these "special" patients do.

Remote rural patients—even those who might not have borderline characters in their own culture's frame of reference—can trigger similar countertransference reactions in urban professional staff. People from remote rural areas often describe themselves as unique, needing special treatment. Furthermore, at least in Alaska, there is a long history of what is perceived as victimization by outsiders. In many families, heavy alcohol abuse is associated with child abuse or child sexual abuse, as well as domestic violence, creating another kind of victimization. Guilt and "overdoing" by treaters, and extreme differences of opinion among treatment staff about individuals as well as whole groups of people, arise frequently. There are no right answers in such situations, but staff can easily become polarized.

Patients often express little gratitude for what has been done, even to those who are "idealized helpers" at some stage in the treatment process. What is being played out in many remote rural situations is an intense, ambivalent mutual attachment between treaters and patients. The psychiatrist needs to be aware of these patterns to avoid getting caught up in interorganizational, interpersonal, or intrapersonal rescuer–victim–bad-guy triangles.

What Can Be Done for the Immediate Problem?

In the case of the former patient who asked for help for her uncle, the senior psychiatrist could refuse to see the patient, could contact the long-haired psychiatrist to talk over the situation, or could offer to consult on the case. Contact with the medical director of the hospital, the immediate supervisor of the long-haired psychiatrist, is also a possibility.

In this case, however, the medical director is a younger person who does not feel comfortable doing administrative work and who is reluctant to be a "bad guy." Therefore, performance appraisals are done in cursory fashion, as is supervision. The long-haired psychiatrist is always rated as excellent so he "won't get mad."

Other possibilities are a brief evaluation of the patient, followed by a referral back to the local psychiatrist, or a second opinion from other local staff.

What Else Could Be Done?

Many of the issues in this and some of the other cases are related to how the personnel system works. Rural health organizations are frequently funded by state or federal monies. Hiring follows bureaucratic personnel guidelines mandated for public programs, and those on the scene may have relatively little control over who is hired and who has privileges at the hospital. Sometimes a "warm-body" philosophy takes hold: A place that has had great difficulty in recruiting, with a job unfilled for a long time, may hire a person who is less than qualified because "a warm body is better than no services at all." Reference checks are sometimes done hastily and inadequately.

Once a person is hired, everyone else may be too swamped to provide a good orientation. Performance appraisals are often done haphazardly by clinical staff who see them as "administrative b.s."

Reforms in the personnel system, greater care in hiring (to the degree it is possible), and considerable attention to orientation of new employees can prevent conflicts caused by doctors with attitude or competence problems. When it can be done, redesigning jobs to promote more interdepartmental and interorganizational linkages can be helpful. Changes might include bridging or linking jobs in which employees work half-time on one staff and half on another, temporary duty details to work with staff in another organization, and increased expectations and incentives in job descriptions and performance appraisals for interdepartmental and interorganizational team efforts.

What Should the Senior Psychiatrist's Role Be?

Work in remote rural areas provides many opportunities for crossed loyalties. Services tend to be provided by public programs because the economics of giving care in these distant sites makes privatizing difficult; the salaried employees are often swamped, with large caseloads and inadequate support staff and facilities. If the employees do not meet everyone's expectations, patients, and sometimes other staff, complain about them and go over their heads to try to fix the problem. If they do perform well, they are apt to be asked to take on all sorts of additional roles, often in conflict with their clinical one. Responsibilities and lines of authority for the extraclinical positions are often unclear.

The senior psychiatrist must be aware of these patterns and must continually try to negotiate greater role clarity. In multilevel systems such as the one described in this case, psychiatrists are frequently asked to function in backup roles. Exactly what the backup role is, however, can be extremely unclear. Because local staff want to retain control of hiring, firing, purchasing, and planning, the person in the backup role has little authority. At the same time, local people often want the backup person to take action or assume responsibility if something goes wrong.

In this case, the senior psychiatrist has no direct or "organizational chart line" authority over the younger one, who works in another facility. Because money does pass from the parent organization to the rural hospital, however, some influence is possible by going up the chain of command in the parent organization and then down the chain of command in the local facility. Because a number of administrators have to be involved in such a process, it is relatively rare for the parent organization to have much say over what happens in individual clinical practices in the field. Yet, even though the "chief" lacks authority, as part of the parent organization, he or she is in theory responsible for seeing that high-quality services are rendered in the field. The senior psychiatrist can muster a certain "organizational energy" through informal communications and relationships that have built up over the years. In this way, it is possible, even without explicit authority, to leverage or influence a situation to move in a certain direction; practically, however, the local leaders have the ultimate say.

Some Advantages and Disadvantages of Remote Rural Psychiatry

There is in the literature and in many people's minds a fairly bleak image of the opportunities and prospects for rural psychiatrists (Jones and Parlour 1985; Pathman et al. 1992; Rabinowitz 1993). For example, it is asserted that psychiatrists may feel frustrated by having to work with physician colleagues who may be somewhat conservative or may hold to the medical model of care. Also, the rural psychiatrist has fewer resources and colleagues available to him or her than the psychiatrist in a metropolitan area. Like psychiatrists in some community mental health centers, rural psychiatrists may see little opportunity for professional growth and may find it hard to work with others who have a social service model or very different values and orientations. Diminished status may be associated with being a public employee (which most rural jobs require), and distrust and resentment of the psychiatrist by nonmedical (or antimedical) mental health center personnel can make him or her feel excluded or marginalized. Lack of backup can leave the psychiatrist overwhelmed, having to be always available to the local nonpsychiatric physicians or mental health staff, to take call every night, to worry about arranging coverage when going on vacation, and so on. Lack of autonomy can also be an issue; the psychiatrist in a remote rural setting may have little control over the kind of work he or she does.

Many feel that training programs do not adequately prepare psychiatrists for rural work. The curriculum, to be relevant and effective for rural practice, would need to include extensive training in such areas as research, program planning, development, management, public health approaches, and community development; it should also include training in working with paraprofessionals, running programs on a shoestring, and dealing with ethical issues integral to treating large volumes of patients without access to the diagnostic and treatment resources available in urban areas. All this would be in addition to psychiatric diagnosis, consultation, and treatment techniques that already fill the curriculum. For rural psychiatrists, there is a dearth of opportunities for continuing education without traveling to distant urban centers at considerable cost in time and money.

Rural psychiatrists and other mental health professionals may feel they are entering a foreign culture, living among a rural population whose attitudes and way of life are entirely new and strange. The culture and the general lack of sophistication are usually quite different from the psychiatrist's own background. In rural areas, newcomers may be perceived as outsiders and often as "youngsters." Locals with a strong sense of self-reliance may be unwilling to seek help. High rates of alcoholism, suicide, and severe behavioral pathology may be difficult to get used to. Proximity to patients and their families can make it difficult for mental health professionals to establish boundaries between their professional and personal activities.

In addition, the psychiatrist's spouse may feel isolated or unable to practice his or her profession because no opportunities are available in the particular rural location. The economic realities of psychiatry in a poor rural area include low salaries and limited opportunities for private practice.

Some, not deterred by the financial and status aspects of rural practice, settle in rural areas but are soon driven away by cultural, professional, and personal isolation. In more than half of all counties in the United States, there are no psychiatrists at all (Langsley and Robinowitz 1979). National Health Service psychiatrists stationed in rural areas usually do not stay on.

Besides the personal, professional, and cultural isolation issues; the economic disincentives; and the proximity to patients, there can be other negatives stemming from the characteristics of the patients. They have probably had few previous professional interventions and therefore do not know what a psychiatrist can offer. In isolated rural settings, patients may be kept at home longer with serious mental problems and may not be brought to the psychiatrist until their problems are extremely hard to treat. Both the most difficult cases and the least challenging ones will be sent to the psychiatrist.

Because the psychiatrist may be the first physician the patient has seen in many years, he or she must look for medical illness and must also be alert for unorthodox treatments given by traditional healers or by general physicians who have been practicing for years in out-of-the-way locations and may now be minimally competent. The psychiatrist may often be left without adequate follow-up for prescribed treatments and may feel frustrated that a treatment that would ordinarily work is blocked because some needed element, easily available elsewhere, is missing.

The psychiatrist may be called on frequently to intervene in high-stress crisis situations and equally frequently to do routine medication checks and "welfare" evaluations for unfamiliar patients. The psychiatrist will be expected to be available at a moment's notice, with constant interruptions.

With long-term chronic patients, staff may not have a realistic conception of what can be accomplished. The passivity and dependency of these patients, and the lack of resources to help them, can lead to staff resentments, especially because in rural settings everyone in the community is highly aware of how patients are doing, including their lack of progress.

For psychiatrists and other mental health professionals who stay in a rural community for a long time, the close personal relationships with local people that develop over the years can create problems. For example, if one has seen a little girl grow up in the community, used her as a baby-sitter for one's own children, seen her in various roles over the years, and known her family, and if she then suicides, or burns to death in a fire, or gets raped, it is a different experience from learning that something similar happened to a person one did not know. In small communities, tragedies have a personal impact on everyone.

Symptoms of burnout can result from any or all of these factors. Such symptoms commonly include the following: 1) decreased job satisfaction, with idealism diminished, enthusiasm down, and disillusionment up; 2) increased negative attitudes and avoidance in relationships with patients; 3) increased irritability in relationships with staff and co-workers; 4) greater discontent with or questioning of the organization's mission and goals; 5) increased irritability in relationship with family; 6) increased exhaustion, apathy, denial, hypomania, physical symptoms, drinking, and negative self-concepts; 7) lower standards, quantity, and quality at work, with increased feelings of being trapped or wanting to leave; and 8) less tolerance for job factors such as time pressures and deadlines, bureaucratic policies and procedures, emotional demands of those seeking services, working conditions, relationship with superiors, peers, and subordinates.

The initial enthusiasm that was felt when starting to work in the rural area and the high hopes, idealism, missionary zeal, and expectation of simple and immediate solutions are no longer present. Instead, various negative attitudes begin to emerge. Feelings of stagnation may lead to doing the job, but wondering, is it worth the effort? Am I paid enough? Could I work fewer hours, or see fewer patients? Is this the best place for me? Am I stalled and losing momentum? Feelings of frustration may be expressed in irritability, challenging both the system and patients, spinning wheels in nonproductive activity, and feeling overwhelmed and confused. Feelings of apathy may result in boredom and detachment, going through the motions, and watching the clock. Feelings of depression and anxiety and psychosomatic complaints are also present to some degree.

This extensive list of potential negatives associated with rural practice can appear rather daunting. It may be even more discouraging to recognize that interprofessional differences can be exacerbated if more than one of those involved are experiencing some of these symptoms. It is therefore important for the psychiatrist and other mental health professionals to be aware of them to anticipate and be prepared for their occurrence.

In contrast to this negative view, however, many professionals have a completely different perspective on working in rural or developing areas, and it is equally important to be aware of the positive and enriching aspects. Living and working in a different or foreign culture can be a challenge and a growth-promoting learning experience, rather than a source of stress and anxiety. Whether the experience is interpreted positively or negatively seems to depend to a great extent on the psychiatrist's professional identity and how it is conceptualized.

In most rural areas, in addition to psychiatrists and physicians, there are professionals of various kinds (e.g., anthropologists, linguists, economists). The close contact with alternative points of view can promote creativity; the psychiatrist is continually forced to question very basic assumptions that would be taken for granted by other mental health professionals. Moreover, computer modems and other evolving forms of communication make a wealth of continuing education material available for home study, and many rural areas are fairly generous with travel funds for training in urban locations. It is possible over time to develop the qualities mentioned in the "job enrichment" literature (Herzberg 1966) in rural jobs. The jobs may involve the following characteristics:

1. Because the jobs can involve a great variety of tasks, it is difficult to get bored. Because a whole portfolio of projects may be in hand, even if one or two are not doing well at any point in time, others are running smoothly and providing satisfaction.
2. There may be frequent changes in the tasks.
3. There is opportunity to identify with and be responsible for a whole piece of work—such as the planning and management, the budgeting, the actual carrying out of the project, and the evaluation—with the satisfactions of accomplishment that can come from successfully completing the project. Younger people many find opportunities to take on the kind of large and complex tasks with substantial responsibility that would be available only to very senior people in urban locations.
4. The jobs may allow for participation in decisions that affect job activities, which allows people to write their own tickets to some extent about the overall work as well as individual projects.
5. The jobs may allow for participation in semiautonomous work groups and teams, in which people from different professions and different cultural groups, who would not otherwise be in such close contact, can learn a great deal from one another.
6. There may be feedback and recognition of performance, because in smaller communities everyone is known and observed. It is possible to see patients or start projects and then keep track of progress for many years.
7. The jobs can provide many opportunities for creativity. The constraints of lack of staff and resources, as well as the occasional lack of theories and program models that fit the particular context, can lead to greater innovation.

Despite inadequate work facilities and other practical problems, work that has these intrinsic characteristics provides tremendous motivation and enjoyment. Rather than feeling marginalized and unappreciated, successful psychiatrists in rural settings learn to value being generalists, becoming skilled in working between disciplines and serving as culture-brokers or shuttle diplomats.

In addition, rural life has some important advantages, including clean air, scenic beauty, opportunities for recreation, less crime and congestion, and a frontier atmosphere where growth and development are under way.

Because psychiatrists are in very short supply in rural areas, the rural psychiatrist can take satisfaction in knowing that he or she is serving a real need. Given the many developing areas of the world that currently lack psychiatric expertise, and the large numbers of immigrants moving from rural to metropolitan areas, skills developed in rural work are likely to be increasingly valued in the future.

To avoid burnout, rural psychiatrists can be sensitive to the early stages described earlier and can take corrective action before the advanced stages set in. This might include planning a vacation or travel to another location, increasing physical exercise, starting a new hobby or project, or other ways to "de-stress" or achieve a change of pace.

If staff members work as a team, frustrations can be dispersed among the individual team members and the team as a whole, rather than overwhelming one individual. A relationship with a difficult set of clients that would become exhausting for the individual professional can be avoided.

The fluidity characteristic of remote rural and frontier settings makes it possible for the professional to build up the lifestyle he or she prefers, often more easily than in a city setting. Alternative part-time activities to build extra income through investments or other means can help compensate for low pay from salaried jobs. As a counterbalance to being perceived by urban professionals as lower in status, there is considerable local status and impact because of the relatively small number of specialists available. Problems of professional isolation can be overcome by building a support network and making active use of various communications possibilities, participating in continuing educational opportunities available through audiocassette, and planning vacations to coincide with professional meetings.

In short, many of the strategies described for dealing with the cases in this book—identifying resources, building support networks, setting clear goals, articulating values, working out a philosophy and priorities, and being creative and flexible in defining one's role—are also effective in avoiding personal feelings of being overwhelmed or burned out.

Recruiting and retention in rural areas require senior people who are enthusiastic about rural opportunities and can mentor younger staff and help them see the positive aspects of the experience, rather than the negatives.

6

Case 5: Help From Granny

The case presented in this chapter illustrates a common problem faced by psychiatrists in remote rural communities. A significant number of people, either in the patient's extended family or in the community as a whole, may have alcohol-related problems. In a small village of 100 people or so, if a few extended families have severe alcohol problems, it can be very difficult to work out aftercare and support for patients returning home to that environment.

A teenage girl who attends high school in an urban area is referred by the school nurse to a psychiatrist for possible depression. She has been very quiet in the classroom and seems rather preoccupied. The psychiatrist sees her only once, because it is almost time for summer break from school.

The girl appears fairly normal to the psychiatrist, although she does seem shy. She does not show signs of major depression, suicidal ideation, or thought disorder. A recent school physical was normal; her school performance is average. She seems to have had a somewhat turbulent relationship with a boyfriend, which recently broke up; the psychiatrist speculates that this event may have caused her current preoccupied behavior. Inquiries about her family back home in the village are met with very brief answers; she admits that there is "a little drinking" in the family and also acknowledges some feelings of homesickness. A cousin has recently died in an alcohol-related drowning back home, but there does not seem to be excessive grief.

The psychiatrist encourages the girl to keep in touch by writing to him once she gets back home, because there has not been time for a full discussion of her situation.

Several weeks later, he receives the following letter from the girl, who is now home in the village:

Dear Dr. X.,

I came home yesterday to the village, and my family wasn't expecting me. One of the men took me home from the airport. When I came into our house, it was a mess. Mom was sleeping, Dad was feeling high, my brother was drinking, and my cousin was also here drinking. My parents had been gambling all night, and when they came home early in the morning, they started drinking. I guess Mom passed out. Dad tried to wake her up after I came in. I threw my junk on my bed and couldn't help crying. My uncle came in drunk also. I came home around 10 A.M. I cleaned up the house, and Mom woke up a couple hours later. Dad went with my uncle to his house to have more booze. Later on my brother left for a ride with his girl. They were out riding all day and came home I think around 8 P.M. Dad and Mom quarreled all day as usual. Dad would turn to me and just bug me. Then he would turn to my younger sister and bug her. Later around 6 P.M. Dad went to my uncle's house again, and Mom went out too. Then around 7 P.M. Dad came in and told me to look for Mom and get her.

My two youngest brothers and I went out, and we went straight to our grandparents' house. That's where we slept, and I came home this morning around 9 A.M. I hated every moment of yesterday. They aren't looking down at me. They're acting the usual. Already people (some) started talking, asking my younger sister why I came home, etc. My cousin kept me company all day yesterday, and we went to church with my grandparents.

Granny told me to sleep at their house every time my parents drink. And that's what I'm going to do. My parents didn't mind when I came in this morning. I told them I'm just fine, except I miss school.

P.S. I talked to Granny and I felt better.

Earlier cases illustrated problems of difficult chronic patients like Dog Bone (Chapter 2), problems of small rural hospitals trying to develop ways to deal with suicidal patients (Chapter 3), problems in which a whole new service program needed to be developed (Chapter 4), and problems that developed when a patient's relative was unhappy with local treatment and wanted to switch doctors (Chapter 5). In the case in this chapter, the psychiatrist must decide how to deal with a dysfunctional family in a distant village.

Is it really possible for a psychiatrist in a remote rural setting to take on the wide range of activities exemplified in these cases? Are there some common patterns that might allow useful skills to be transferred from one kind of situation to another? Or is there so much difference between, say, a hospital system and a family system that it is better for psychiatrists to limit their activities and "just say no" when extraclinical problems come up?

Analyzing a Family System

After getting the girl's letter, the psychiatrist realized that he had not obtained a lot of key information about the family during his brief assessment. Even though he did not have enough information for a full genogram, however, he found it helpful to begin to sketch out the family, using a diagram (Figure 6–1).

From a remote rural perspective, there are several things to try to highlight in such a diagram (Francis 1988; Goodluck 1988; Hartman 1978; Heinl 1985, 1987; McGoldrick and Gerson 1985; Mead et al. 1993;

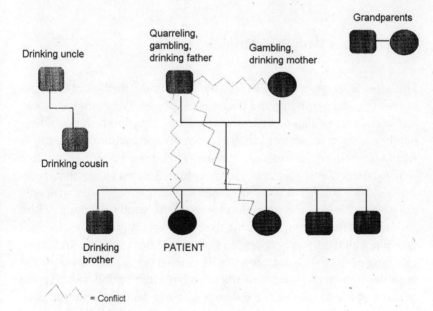

Figure 6–1. Initial family system information.

Minuchin 1981, 1982). It is most important to identify those family members who appear to be functioning well. In this case, it is the grandparents, and possibly the younger brothers. Since resources are scarce, these family members may need to be involved as "cotherapists" to help support the patient. In addition, it appears that there are at least seven people who need help: uncle, cousin, parents, brother, sister, as well as the patient. The three younger children in the family are in high-risk situations and should probably be involved in prevention programming.

Extended Families

Genograms have been drawn to attempt to identify everyone in typical extended families in Alaskan villages. Some of these have 90 or more members, most of whom live in the same community. The family in this case probably includes many people that the psychiatrist has not learned about yet. Because of the intimate living arrangements in a village, where everyone comes into contact with everyone else daily, there are apt to be both further problems to be uncovered and a range of people who could be supportive if the situation could be better assessed.

Environments With High Drinking Levels

The letter describes a family in which mother and father are both drinking heavily and gambling, and the house is a "mess." A brother, an uncle, and a cousin are also described as drinking. The situation is unfortunately common in remote rural Alaskan villages, where frequently a whole community is drinking. A plane (sometimes known locally as a "booze bomber") brings alcohol supplies to an isolated village that is otherwise "dry." The whole town may then start drinking heavily, with only the young children and possibly a teacher or devoutly religious person abstaining. The drinking lasts until the bottles are emptied. This does not take place all the time, because alcohol is often not available. Treatment planning needs to take into account the impact of possible heavy-drinking environments on follow-up and aftercare. From a public health point of view, trying to change the community-wide drinking patterns is essential; it is difficult to help individuals when the drinking level in the rest of the community is so high.

Social Networks

Social network therapy has been a seldom used but widely lauded approach to the treatment of mental and emotional disturbances. The President's Commission on Mental Health (1978) stated as one of its national goals:

> The personal and social supports which currently exist in our neighborhoods and communities are one of the great resources in American society for maintaining mental health and for preventing the development of serious mental and emotional disabilities. Families, friends, neighbors, schools, religious institutions, self-help groups, and voluntary associations are the individuals and kinds of organizations to which most of us initially turn when we have problems. We need to enhance their ability to contribute to the mental health of friends, neighbors, and families. (p. 10)

Cutler and Madore (1980), as well as others, emphasized the importance of social networks in the development and maintenance of mental health and described the need to build a new, permanent "family-like group" for mentally ill persons who have exhausted their "natural kin networks." His work is similar to that of Speck and Attneave (1973) and Ruvinni (1978); one difference is that most of the networks he works with are made up of community agency persons as opposed to natural kin, friends, neighbors, and work associates. The intent, however, is to involve as much of the potential network in the community as can be found.

Social network approaches may be more feasible in small rural communities than in larger cities.

Epidemiological Studies

In other locations, extensive work has been done on the whole question of social and community support networks. Leighton et al. (1963a), for example, studied the effects of blocked strivings in several Canadian maritime communities in Nova Scotia. Known as the Stirling County study, the research correlated the degree of psychiatric disorder with social disintegration. Leighton et al. argued that disintegrated communities interfere with the vital strivings of individuals. Conversely, disordered individuals are not effective in creating integrated communities, nor do they raise their children in ways conducive to learning successful coping modes.

Other studies have been done on the links between community integration and mental health in non-Western societies. Leighton collaborated with Lambo, a Nigerian psychiatrist, and others in a study of social epidemiology of the Yoruba of Nigeria (Leighton et al. 1963b). Using the same methods as in the Stirling County study, they got similar results. Yoruba men and women were at greatest risk of psychiatric impairment, judged in terms of Western psychiatry, if they lived in more disintegrated communities.

Obstacles to Family and Social Network Therapy

A case like the one considered here can present several problems from the psychiatric point of view. One is how to get a good family history in the first place, especially when the time available for assessment is very brief. Unless good rapport can be established, a history of substance abuse in the extended family may be missed or minimized.

In remote rural areas, it is also important to learn as much as possible about those members of the family who are doing well but who may be mentioned only in passing unless specific inquiries are made; in this case, these are the grandparents, and possibly other relatives the psychiatrist has not yet heard about. Lack of professional resources may mean that such family members will be "cotherapists" whom the psychiatrist will need to encourage and work with.

With prevention or early treatment in mind, the psychiatrist in this case would also try to find out more about the two younger brothers, who may be at high risk for future problems if nothing is done, as well as the younger sister, who is being "bugged" by the alcoholic father.

Cutler and Madore (1980) described one way to get family information more easily. Assessments are done on the families, and family records are filed under each head of household. Progress notes are entered sequentially in the chart as family, marital, individual, or group therapy contacts with family members. This policy forces the worker to think of the family as the basic social unit.

Another problem, as in this case, is that an urban psychiatrist may not be familiar with the particular rural community to which the patient will return and may not know what resources are available there. Thus, even if a good assessment has been possible while the patient is in the city, the psychiatrist must consider what kind of treatment approach can be worked out once the patient returns home to a remote rural community.

A related, and extremely common, problem in settings like Alaska is that patients who are evaluated in big cities often receive brief treatment there. They usually do well while in the structured treatment settings with intensive specialized care. However, they then go home to a remote village that has minimal or nonexistent aftercare or follow-up services; those for teenagers and children are in especially short supply. In addition, some villages are extremely dysfunctional, with large numbers of heavy alcohol users not only in the family but in the rest of the community.

This case is representative of a large number of difficult therapeutic situations in which children are being raised in heavy-drinking environments and are in remote communities where access to professional treatment is minimal.

The Urban Villager

This case also provides an example of the increasingly common phenomenon of "urban villagers." These are people who move back and forth between small rural communities and larger cities and who keep many of their values and behaviors from village life even when in the city. Problems can arise, for example, for a patient who moves into the city to try to sober up and get away from heavy-drinking relatives. When the relatives come to town to visit, the patient feels tremendous pressure to start drinking again. The urban psychiatrist treating people with rural roots must be aware of each patient's background; a large number of rural people, including immigrants and refugees, now live in large cities, and the kinship ties can be surprisingly strong.

Who "Owns" the Problem?

In rural areas, patients like this teenage girl often get bounced back and forth among various agencies—substance abuse programs, mental health programs, the school system, and sometimes child protection services—without finding much help or support. Many substance abuse programs are not skilled at dealing with depression or doing family counseling, and Al-Anon, Alateen, Adult Children of Alcoholics, and other Alcoholics Anonymous types of programs are often not organized in small rural villages. Mental health programs, on the other hand, may not deal very well with substance abuse problems. The schools generally do not know what to do. Child welfare workers, swamped with heavy caseloads, tend to focus on younger children with clear-cut physical or sexual abuse. Girls like this one, who are older, somewhat shy and non-verbal, and more neglected than abused, are unlikely to be removed from their homes. The family members, who could also be considered as owning the problem, are apt to be in a state of denial. The community as a whole, despite considerable effort by public agencies to encourage "community ownership" of problems, may not be able to organize much of a response.

This girl is at high risk for continued problems, such as teen pregnancy, sexual abuse, dropping out of school, substance abuse, and suicidal behavior. Other children in the family are also at risk.

Assembling All the Part-Owners

The girl in this case does have some resources—her grandparents, possibly the church, people at her school, other relatives, the psychiatrist—who might be considered part-owners of the problem. Ideally, all these resources will be assembled to help her cope with a very difficult family situation. A larger question is whether a response can be formulated that would be helpful across the board, so that the many remote rural communities where children are being raised in heavy-drinking environments can develop local capacity to deal with the problems.

What Can Be Done for the Immediate Problem?

Organizing From a Distance

To identify the resources available in the girl's community will probably require some long-distance phone calls to the regional programs (substance abuse, mental health) and possibly to the village. A table of potential resources like Table 2–1 (Chapter 2) can be helpful; no possible people or programs should be left out. A phone call directly to the girl to assess the situation and discuss options with her, or a reply to her letter, might then be in order.

There may be relatively little available at the village level, and even itinerant regional workers may not be able to offer much. In that case, periodic brief phone calls from the psychiatrist can provide some support, helping the patient cope with a difficult situation until she returns to school. It is possible to conduct long-distance "telephone rounds" to keep up contact with a number of patients, or with cotherapists or service providers in the village whom the psychiatrist is backing up. Brief letters to patients in remote settings can also be extremely effective in providing support.

The psychiatrist should be aware of possible problems in employing this strategy, however. For one thing, there may be no telephone in the village or only one public phone that provides no privacy for the caller.

There are also legal issues to consider. A psychiatrist who is dealing with a high-risk patient at a considerable distance has little ability to control what happens. The psychiatrist does not want to abandon a patient, but a continuing relationship maintained by phone calls and letters is less than ideal. If the patient has a crisis while in the remote community, and there are no local people actively involved, the psychiatrist is at some risk of being held legally responsible for any resulting problems.

Some ethical questions may arise as well. Is it better to keep up some supportive contact with patients like this, who will otherwise not have access to professional help? Or is it better for them to cope as best they can on their own, getting help from "Granny" or others when they can? If there are regional midlevel providers, the psychiatrist must also decide whether to play a direct role or to provide backup from a distance.

Setting Priorities

Given the psychiatrist's limited time and the large number of patients like this, another question is how to get the most results. Is the time best spent in functioning as a clinician, trying to set up a regional clinic to see some of these teenagers? Would a family counseling approach work better than seeing individuals? Or would it be better to spend the time trying to develop local capacity, encouraging elders-youth projects; grand-mothers' clubs; youth support groups and "natural helpers" or peer counselor types of programs; Al-Anon, Alateen, and Adult Children of Alcoholics programs; and other self-help and paraprofessional efforts?

Providing backup to such programs by telephone or periodically in person raises problems similar to those encountered in giving long-distance support directly to the patient. The psychiatrist has little ability to control what is done at a distant site. On the other hand, the costs of providing intensive professional services in these remote rural communities can be prohibitive, and the professional who does visit the site may soon feel that nothing but "putting on Band-Aids" is possible because the family conditions are likely to create high-risk youth faster than the current cases can be handled.

Developing Local Capacity

A major effort is under way in Alaska to develop village capacity to deal with alcoholic families. Paraprofessional village counselor positions have been established, as well as regional teen substance abuse outreach and aftercare coordinators. Specialized training, including creation of curricula and training manuals, university-based efforts to get certification systems in place, and statewide and regional workshops, is being developed to give village paraprofessionals and regional backup teams the skills they need to work with adolescents and their families. Difficult problems that in urban locations would be handled by subspecialists will in remote rural areas be dealt with by paraprofessionals and mid-level staff.

Network Approaches

The purpose of the family network therapy approach is to ensure that all participating family members and agency persons are involved in solving the problem. The assumption is that the problem is as much a function of the context in which it occurs as of the person with the problem behavior. Therefore, the participation of all those who make up the social and family context is crucial to evaluating and processing the family members' individual problems. The inclusion of all agencies as well as extended family members prevents the agencies from competing with one another and from colluding to scapegoat particular family members. Finally, family members, observing their own participation and that of the agency people, begin to feel there is hope if everyone can work together.

However, network therapy cannot be done routinely because of the large expenditure in human resources and time needed. It can be best used when:

1. A crisis state exists and is continuing to expand with no indications that a spontaneous resolution will occur.
2. Increasing distress within the family is producing symptoms in more than one member.
3. Multiple contacts with many agencies are yielding little or no results.
4. Temporary or permanent removal of the symptomatic family member is deemed impossible or not helpful.
5. Family members and staff view the problem as potentially disastrous without a major overhaul.
6. Lack of interagency coordination exacerbates communication problems, thus adding to the blaming process.
7. Agency workers feel discouraged or believe that they are dealing with a "hopeless" family.

Sometimes a network organizer helps carry out network therapy. This must be someone who is well known, trusted, and respected and who has contacts with people at many levels in the community; an outsider would not be able to fill this role. Other participants may include 1) an advocate for each family member (similar to a double in psychodrama), 2) a conductor to keep things moving and focused until a "network effect" (in which people start to work better as a group) develops, 3) consultants, and 4) a monitor to be sure there is follow-through on agreed-on treatment plans by all concerned.

Billing for a network approach can sometimes be worked out; it can be made clear to funding sources that these families can otherwise cost tremendous amounts in terms of staff and agency time.

In very remote rural settings with extremely limited resources, a well-staffed, formal network approach is generally not possible. However, the psychiatrist can use the same type of thinking and see that similar types of approach, usually on a scaled-down and less comprehensive basis, are carried out.

What Else Could Be Done?

In rural Alaska, a number of different methods are being tried in an attempt to strengthen family values and encourage communities to change social norms about drinking.

Translating Terms and Concepts

One such effort involves identifying terms and concepts in the local languages that are related to family counseling. There is considerable variation, and it is interesting to hear Yupik Eskimos' comments on Iñupiaq descriptions, for example, during discussions of similarities and differences in how families are perceived and how both groups compare with majority-culture families.

Not much is known about how extended family systems from these specific cultural groups work. Some concepts seem to translate fairly well between Eskimo and English, whereas others do not. It is hoped that preparation of specialized mental health dictionaries and glossaries to describe the local cultural constructs will lead to a better understanding of how to be helpful. Such materials should be useful in health education efforts, in discussions with elders about how they can help their children, and in orientation of new non-Native health professionals coming into the remote rural area.

Strengthening Cultural Identity

Another effort, which has won national recognition, is the Spirit Program in the Kotzebue region (Craig 1988; McNabb 1991), in which elders work with youth in many different ways (e.g., elders-youth workshops, special school programs, culture camps, regional heroes programs, revitalization of traditional ceremonial activities, language preservation, radio and television educational efforts). Most of the communities in this region have active village councils and have "voted dry" under a local-option alcohol law. In one village, elders are helping to design a new school curriculum; they feel that part of the problem stems from youth losing touch with their cultural values and roots because of an overly "white" school system. Elders come into the schools as role models and mentors. One example of change is that seals or caribou, important elements of the Native culture, may be dissected in biology courses instead of nonlocal frogs.

Tribal Family Courts

Another community has set up a tribal court in which elders and other village leaders meet to discuss community problems. Under federal treaties with American Indian and Alaska Native tribes, a tribal organization may set up its own legal system. The tribal courts can choose to take on most of the same functions that state courts would, especially with regard to civil matters occurring on tribal lands.

When a child is being abused or neglected by an alcoholic family, the tribal court can give warnings to the parents. If the warnings are not heeded, the child can be removed from the home to stay with relatives, and the parents are required to go to a residential center for treatment of their substance abuse problems. To keep treatment costs down, and to make it easier for rural parents who are not used to big cities, the residential treatment is carried out in a remote "fish-camp" setting. People at the camp must do chores (e.g., fish, hunt, gather firewood) as well as receive counseling, generally from paraprofessionals and through self-help groups.

If the tribal court approach is rejected by the family, the state authorities can be asked to institute formal legal proceedings to remove the child from the parents' custody. This is a last resort, however. Community members make every effort to handle the problem through their own social control methods, such as peer-group pressure and use of volunteers.

Changing Community Norms

Some small communities, working for more than 20 years, have made major strides in "re-norming" the whole community. Most urban psychiatrists, experienced with big-city community mental health efforts, would be skeptical about this possibility. But an isolated, remote village, with a population of 75–100 people, is an entirely different kind of community from the city "community catchment" area of 75,000 people or more.

There are a number of success stories of small communities that have not only voted dry and enforced it, but slowly changed the community norms so that alcohol use and related behaviors are not tolerated. Such communities have been able to articulate their values and create productive, "therapeutic" communities through methods reminiscent of the "moral treatment" of an earlier era.

Once a community sobers up, a host of other structural problems usually remain (e.g., lack of jobs, chronic health problems resulting from the former alcohol abuse, unresolved grief reactions). A community in Canada (Alkali Lake) has made some moving documentaries about the stages it went through in its community-wide recovery process. Voting dry is just a beginning step in the long-term development effort that is needed for recovery.

Early Intervention Efforts

A variety of early intervention efforts are also under way in Alaska to set up programs for young children and their families before the children become problem teenagers. These include programs in prenatal clinics to identify and offer special counseling for high-risk substance-abusing families, "home start" programs to help young parents with parenting, "home builders" and in-village family treatment efforts, and Head Start "family wellness" projects. From a prevention or early intervention point of view, the girl in this case is coming to the psychiatrist's attention about 14 years too late!

What Should the Psychiatrist's Role Be?

In this case, like others in this book, the psychiatrist might take on a variety of extraclinical roles, ranging from developer of professional training systems to linguist and medical anthropologist to backup provider for local counselors. Numerous different approaches to the problem may involve the psychiatrist in the planning and design of health education efforts; the development of programs targeted at high-risk groups; needs assessment and other data-gathering efforts; and, perhaps most importantly, helping to change alcohol laws by providing testimony to legislators, writing position papers, and working with lobbyists retained by professional organizations.

Although the psychiatrist working in remote rural areas may not feel prepared to take on all of these roles, he or she must at least be aware of them as part of the overall picture. The psychiatrist can then consult with local grant writers or other appropriate people to search for ways to use local talent or to build new resources into the local system. In other words, an expanded awareness of what *could* be happening will help the psychiatrist sense what is missing and will also help prevent a business-as-usual approach that overlooks opportunities and needs in remote rural settings. The average clinician, for instance, does not usually consider adding an anthropologist or linguist or paraprofessional training officer to a treatment team. In certain remote rural settings, however, these roles can contribute a lot to program capacity.

Goal Setting

The basic principle is to have a clear vision of "what could be" and then to compare it with "what is." The creative tension that results can provide the impetus for innovative ideas. Dealing only with "what is" can lead to a circumscribed, crisis-oriented approach. Dealing only with "what could be" can lead to vague idealism. A balance between the two can stimulate effective program development.

Network Therapy and the Psychiatrist's Role

As mentioned earlier, Cutler and Madore's (1980) approach uses a network organizer, an advocate for each family member, a conductor, consultants, and a monitor to track progress on treatment agreements. It would be highly unusual for a remote rural psychiatrist to have so many ancillary personnel. The same basic approach, however, can often be used if the psychiatrist is able to assemble a team of local paraprofessionals and regional backup staff.

The staff doing the network therapy try to create an attitudinal setting for a cooperative, active, problem-solving experience, even if family members who are initially resistant to the procedure try to lay blame or scapegoat, feel attacked, get angry, feel discouraged, lose self-esteem, or feel victimized. Family members must redefine their roles with respect to one another. Assessments reveal how the members define the problem and perceive their own needs in relation to the family system. At times the family is not ready to change or can make only a limited degree of change.

No matter what the outcome for the family, the community benefits from a greater knowledge of the problem's depth and longevity; increased understanding of roles, functions, and goals among persons as well as agencies; a reduction of energy wasting; and added respect and common experience among staff of collaborating agencies.

Developing collaboration and opportunities for consultation with a variety of community agencies has obvious primary and secondary preventative implications. Linkages resulting from the network approach have provided jumping-off points for collaborative efforts between family guidance clinics and other agencies in developing a wide range of programs. Nitty-gritty, frontline involvement is very powerful in establishing trust among the agencies and has an important staff development function.

Community network therapy is not meant to be a cure-all. It is designed to open lines of communication between family members and significant community persons and to keep them open to prevent further dissolution and crisis and to facilitate positive efforts for all family members and agency persons. It gives staff an in vivo perspective in working within the context from which mental and emotional problems emerge. Because it takes time, it cannot be used in every case, but it can be cost effective if used to handle problem families that would otherwise be highly resistant to change and would consume large amounts of staff time.

Another Point of View

In multicultural situations, it can be instructive to hear comments from local cultural mentors, using terms and concepts in the local language, to see whether their analysis of interview material matches that of the professionals. The degree of mismatch between the psychiatrist's formulation and that of the local informant can suggest areas that should be explored further. The following is an Iñupiaq Eskimo's perspective on the case.

An Iñupiaq View of the Problem

The parents have decided not to live. They are denying their responsibility for living. They want to live for now, in an irresponsible way, and forget about their responsibilities as parents, and about tomorrow.

The children are victims of their "dysfunctional" family. They have a chance of becoming alcoholic or marrying into an alcoholic family themselves. Their best hope would be a "Concerns Committee," or local village task force, with elders, church members, and so on, from the village. This committee could talk over what should be done to intervene and help make decisions on behalf of the children. They could talk with the welfare worker and decide if foster homes might be needed, and how to encourage the girl to return to school.

There appear to be no resources for family support in the village. The village alcohol program is not being responsive. The school, the village coordinator, and the outreach staff are not mentioned. The problems may therefore escalate, unless a village "Concerns Committee" is functioning, until someone breaks down mentally or dies or someone gets institutionalized.

There are several Eskimo terms and concepts that would apply in this family situation.

1. *Iqsiqi.* This term means "fear." The children have this and probably the grandparents.
2. *Piagtuggi.* This term means "abuse." The parents are abusive of their family.
3. *Nakungitchuk.* This term means "he or she is unwell." We have a different expression when the whole family unit is not well, or is sick, or not okay, which is *kitungagiit nakungitchat.*
4. *Tutqiitch.* The girl is "ill at ease," or *tutqiitch,* and can't get comfortable because it's not a healthy, safe place.
5. *Qiniq, ummisuk.* The father, and maybe both parents, as well as the son that is drinking, probably have a remorseful mood of anger, which we term *qiniq.* This term describes a type of angry pouting, which results from a certain frame of mind where one cannot step out of the situation. One is "stuck" being angry—a condition known as *ummisuk.* To get out of this stage, it will take talking, prayer, and listening.
6. *Alliasuk, allianiiq, qivit.* The girl seems depressed (*alliasuk*) and lonely (*allianiiq*). It might take only a short time for her to *qivit,* a term

that refers to letting go of hope. One stops cleaning up the house, becomes the opposite of a concerned person, more an uncaring person, and can be at high risk for being suicidal.

What could be done?   From an Iñupiaq point of view, there are some basic values that relate to respect for others; this includes ideas about noninterference. A Native counselor might spend a considerable time with people in this family, appearing to a non-Native to be doing nothing. The counselor is available but, out of respect, does not rush in with a quick fix or intervene in a way that might cause additional conflict. Avoidance of conflict is one of our traditional values. This has been misinterpreted by some who have written about it as a form of fatalism. It is actually based on ideas of respect that have proven highly adaptive over thousands of years.

Besides close observation, noninterference, respect for all people involved, and avoidance of conflict, a view of the problem as a group or communal one is likely for a Native counselor. Solutions such as asking a village "Concerns Committee" to work on the problem might not immediately occur to a non-Native counselor. In a big city, there would be more focus on individual treatment by professionals; in a small village, the collective approach is more feasible. Traditional Iñupiat culture emphasizes following a path based on values. It would be helpful if non-Native counselors became more familiar with these ideas, rather than being so quick to try to fit us into non-Native diagnostic labels and categories. There are several important concepts.

1. *Nalluat, nallungnga, nalluanngaitch, nalu.*   These terms deal with "rightness" and "not rightness." *Nalluat* is right in the sense of "you've hit the bull's-eye" or "you're doing the best thing you could do or making the best decision." It deals more with specific situations. *Nallungnga* is a more general term, meaning that everything is in focus and being done right or in a positive way. *Nalluanngaitch* means that things are not right or that everything is "out of whack." *Nalu* is a term for "not knowing."

   The sophisticated psychology here involves ideas about consciousness, following a positive spiritual path, and not getting stuck in unhealthy patterns. In this case, the parents are drinking, not communicating, giving up on life, and "not doing the right thing."

   The girl would have a feeling of being stuck and may soon no longer have the option of going back to school. Her mental feelings of "stuckness" will soon tend to lead actually to being trapped—getting into the same cycle her parents are in of drinking, having children early, dropping out of school, and so on.

The girl is trying to "do the right thing" by talking, writing letters, continuing her relationship with her grandmother, and reaching out to people, rather than isolating herself. She is trying to stay in school, rather than dropping out; to marry, rather than being promiscuous; and to choose life and stay sober, rather than suiciding or becoming an alcoholic.

Her path has two different ways to go. If she enters the state of *nalu* or not knowing, the "right" side of the path will be forgotten and out of her awareness, and all she will see is the negative.

Allapit is a related term that refers to a lack of consciousness, "no knowledge," or "everything is black." It is also sometimes translated as "forgetfulness." Again, this term is about diverting attention or paying no attention to what is going on. People suffering from this condition could get "lost" in the sense that ambition would decrease, as would motivation and sense of identity. It does not take long for the psyche and sense of aliveness to start to die.

2. *Kanaqsriliq.* This term refers to "honoring" or to "being obedient." It could refer to obeying in the sense of completing one's studies on time, or to the honor of being a woman and getting married and having children. It involves mental discipline. This term also refers to following a path based on values.

3. *Ukpik, ukpigingitch.* This term means "to believe." The opposite term would be *allapisaaq* or diverting attention, not listening, diverting interest or priorities. When you divert attention, it is the opposite of "to believe." If I do not believe or do not follow the instructions of a teacher, or someone's directions, it could also be said that I am *ukpigingitch.*

4. *Alqaqsri.* This is a term for someone who gives discipline or lays down the law. This would be done not by just saying what should be done, but by discussing the choices that a person has; the possible consequences of following the right path, based on awareness, consciousness, and group values; and the possible consequences of following the wrong path, being disobedient, disrespectful, unaware, and forgetful.

These concepts are part of a rich, well-thought-out psychology that shares much with Asian psychologies; all are based on ideas of a spiritual path, respect, awareness, close observation of experience, avoidance of conflict, and many related ideas. Psychology and spiritual practices are seen as connected, because clear consciousness, openness, and awareness are needed for spiritual work. Although "mental events" are part of this psychology, there is less emphasis on the individual than in Western psychologies and more concentration on spiritual states that lead to transcendence, going beyond self-centered concerns and identifying with the greater needs of the tribe and higher powers.

Many traditional practices reinforced these values. For example, teaching stories told children what happened to the child who observed and listened to the elders and to other children who did not listen or respect the teachings of elders and wound up suffering as a result. Ceremonies were held at times such as when the young boy killed his first animal. The meat was shared, with the best pieces being given to elders. Such practices reinforced values about sharing, putting the survival of the group above individual needs, and respecting elders for their greater experience.

When non-Natives came in, they brought a very different value system that emphasizes competition and looking out for number one; psychological treatments are based on very different assumptions about what a psyche is, the role of spirituality, and how feelings like anger should be channeled.

Many of today's problems seem to be the reverse of our traditional values—child abuse instead of respect for family members, violence instead of avoidance of conflict, and alcoholic blackouts instead of awareness and close observation of experience. The longer-term solutions seem to call for a reaffirmation of our traditional values and development of ways to transmit them to our children, adapting the teachings to modern times.

Psychiatrists could be helpful, if there are attempts to understand us on our own terms. Coming out to conduct psychiatric clinics or medication checks may be of some help for emergencies, but it is very limited compared with the depth of understanding and degree of collaboration with local people that are really needed.

For example, in extended families, there are different kinds of relationships; a person goes to certain relatives for advice about certain types of problems. Family therapists need a better understanding of these dynamics, from an Eskimo point of view, before rushing in to try to do family therapy. Also, there are considerable differences between cultural groups and even between coastal and inland villages in which people speak the same language. Lumping everyone together as Natives, and then trying to help them with off-the-shelf approaches developed for other cultures, is not too satisfactory.

Modern technology can help describe and disseminate these traditional values; a "back-to-the-blanket" approach is not being recommended. Multimedia computer technology can be used to develop interactive computer-assisted instruction. This could be helpful to Native youth, as well as for orientation for non-Native health professionals. We are developing school programs, summer camps, elders-youth conferences, and other projects to build increased awareness of these values.

Training Workshop for Native Counselors

The following account demonstrates how the case of the teenage girl was used in a workshop for Native alcohol counselors. The methods and techniques can be adapted for work with other cultural groups, or for training paraprofessionals and midlevel practitioners. This training session was conducted by an Iñupiaq Eskimo who is highly regarded for her ability to incorporate traditional ideas into her presentations. The subject was problems of aftercare and follow-up when alcohol treatment clients seen in cities return home to their villages. Most of the 15 counselors at the workshop had themselves grown up in villages, but they now worked in various regions in the state.

The approach used by the trainer is experiential, with lots of audience participation. It uses terms and language familiar to the trainees and attempts to weave together various types of information, building on a general philosophical framework. It might be called a "psychophilosophy" (defined later) and is related as much as possible to firsthand personal experiences of the trainees, rather than being objectified and impersonal.

The training session was begun by a male Native counselor who worked in a regional alcohol treatment center, who explained that his program was beginning to incorporate traditional Native values into client activities, including group exercises for each value. For example, the value of "knowledge of family tree" had workbook-type exercises. When the clients had all attempted to reconstruct their own network of family relations, there were group discussions about family values, generational conflicts, how the family impacted on their drinking behavior, and so on. This was felt to be more effective with their cultural group than the Alcoholics Anonymous type of group meetings, although these were also carried out.

The trainer then asked the group to form two lines facing each other. After learning the words, each person had to introduce him- or herself to the others in Iñupiaq. In another group exercise, illustrating the value of humor, one line of participants had to make the other side laugh, while the other side was to stay serious for as long as possible. This exercise evoked responses ranging from telling of jokes to making funny faces and considerable loosening up of what had been a very serious session. Still another exercise asked participants to think of an image expressing how they felt about their role and their relationship with others. For example, one person felt like a "dumb salmon," swimming up- and downstream each year. Another felt like a blueberry: "I get stepped on and squashed, but there are a whole lot of us!"

At this point, the participants moved their chairs into a circle, and the trainer began reading the teenage girl's case. Although the case might not seem very moving to professionals from another culture, a number of trainees were near tears by the end. It triggered many associations in people's minds to experiences they had had themselves when growing up.

The trainer then asked the group to suggest ways that, as counselors, they might try to help this girl with an aftercare plan. The audience called out their answers, which were listed on a chart. At first, the answers were rather conventional and focused on individual work with the girl. As time went on, there was consideration of how other family members and supports from within the community might be encouraged. The recommendations, listed in the order they were suggested, included the following:

- Provide support.
- Do not be judgmental of the family.
- Educate her about alcohol.
- Continue the psychiatrist's support by letter.
- Affirm her choice to stay at grandparents' or another place if grandparents not available.
- Encourage her to do good things each day.
- Explain to her she's not responsible for her parent's action.

- Help her make a choice whether to stay at home or return to school (if she stays home, she'll get stuck in the same patterns as her family).
- Have a professional educate the family. (There was considerable discussion on this point; some felt an "outside expert" would not be able to form a relationship with the family.)
- Get the girl to attend Alateen.

The trainer then gave some of her own comments on the case, using Iñupiaq terms and English translations, with extensive interweaving of other experiential types of material. For example, to illustrate the ideas in Iñupiat psychology about being attentive and having conscious awareness, she recalled the exercise of trying to make other people laugh and explained that the mental state at the moment a person forgot to be serious and laughed instead was what was being referred to by one of the Iñupiaq terms. A number of stories illustrated other psychological aspects of the case that counselors needed to be aware of in order to be helpful.

Some of the participants spoke Yupik Eskimo, a different language from Iñupiaq. They were quite interested in this discussion and tried to think of equivalent terms in Yupik to what the trainer described for Iñupiaq words and concepts.

Interspersed with this discussion was much information about other related projects (e.g., elders-youth school programs, efforts to learn from tribal doctors). The counselors were thus exposed to a wealth of information loosely organized around themes in the case. Various visual teaching tools were used, including the poster reproduced in Figure 6–2; developed as part of an effort to improve Iñupiat self-esteem, it is a succinct expression of basic values and beliefs. There were comments about the role of language, impacts of the school system, the role of the church, transgenerational issues involving the grandparents, and so on.

Case histories like the teenage girl's can be interwoven with descriptions of program activities, group exercises that stress active participation and observation of one's own experience, terms in the local language, and teaching stories. Because the cases include experiences similar to those of other people from the culture, they can seem more real and carry a power that might not be obvious at first to people not from the culture. What is communicated, especially when Native role models lead the discussion, might be termed a psychophilosophy—a therapeutic approach that helps people reconnect with cultural values and deal with identity issues that are seen as root problems.

Every Iñupiaq is responsible to all other Inupiat for
the survival of our cultural spirit, and the values
and traditions through which it survives.
Through our extended family, we retain,
teach, and live our Iñupiaq way.

With guidance and support from Elders,
We Must Teach our children Iñupiaq values:

Knowledge of Language
Sharing
Respect for Others
Cooperation
Respect for Elders
Love for Children
Hard Work
Knowledge of Family Tree
Avoidance of Conflict
Respect for Nature
Spirituality
Humor
Family Roles
Hunter Success
Domestic Skills
Humility
Responsibility to Tribe

Our understanding of our universe and
our place in it is a belief in God and
a respect for all his creations.

Figure 6–2.   Iñupiaq values.

Examples From Other Settings

The examples given here expand on various aspects of the "Granny" case, particularly the need to take varying family and cultural values into consideration.

Alzheimer's Patient From Appalachia

An Alzheimer's patient, accompanied by her adult daughter, goes to an urban teaching hospital (Halperin 1994). During the hospital stay, both the young resident and the attending physician put great pressure on the daughter to place her mother in a nursing home. The family is originally from Appalachia but has recently moved to the city.

Although the mother is increasingly incontinent, disoriented, and at times combative and difficult to handle, her daughter will not consider a nursing home. To place her mother in such a home would be like "putting her away" in a prison.

After much discussion of the intergenerational ties that are keystones of Appalachian social structure and the deeply felt idea that placement of elderly relatives in nursing homes is the near equivalent of a death sentence, home nursing care and an Alzheimer's day care center for 3 days each week are considered by the health care team. The patient returns home where she can be cared for by her daughter and two neighbors, a mother and her adult daughter. In addition, "grandma" receives love and attention from her great-grandchildren. She spends a great deal of time on her front porch overlooking the neighborhood and also spends several days each month with her other daughter and her grown children.

A Bedouin Father

A traditional Bedouin man has fathered 26 children and is negotiating for another wife to continue to add to his family (Bernard 1988). Local clinicians indicate that several of his children had a "failure to thrive" syndrome resulting from undernutrition. Yet the presence of foreign guests prompts the presentation of an extravagant meal, creating the appearance of affluence.

In situations where traditional cultural values are strongly held, professionals have to consider interventions that may take two or three generations to succeed. In this case, there may be few viable incentives to change the personal priorities of the Bedouin host. However, with sufficient external incentives, persuading him to allow his children to continue in school might be possible, although he views schooling as having little value. If this can be done, the children are likely to outdistance him in terms of psychological modernity. It is important to seek change in those areas that pose the least challenge to core cultural ideas and then to build in steps to encompass more central aspects of health-relevant activity. This process requires trust as well as visible and valued outcomes.

A Mexican American Family

This case illustrates Cutler and Madore's (1980) use of family network therapy; his work is well worth reading in its entirety. The approach has common features with the one described in this book, but it is more organized, using different staff in roles of network organizer, advocates for individual family members, and monitors to track progress over time.

The wife in this case is 36 years old and has recurrent bouts of bipolar disorder. Currently on lithium, she has had six hospitalizations for her psychiatric illness. Her husband is an alcoholic, 36-year-old miner. He has been having an affair with another woman who is now 8½ months pregnant.

The four children in the family all have significant problems. A boy age 14 and a girl age 11 are both said by the schoolteacher and counselor to be "mentally retarded and emotionally disturbed." Both are doing poorly in school, are easily distracted and discouraged, and have begun to steal. The girl is friendly but functions at only the third-grade level in school. Both children fight constantly with each other and with the younger children. The 4-year-old boy is frequently in trouble with the neighbors and with family members; he destroys other children's toys and recently set fire to a mattress in the house. The 18-month-old girl appears to be an "undernourished milk baby," according to the local public health nurse. The parents blame each other for the family's problems, and a divorce appears to be pending.

The network organizer contacted and assembled approximately

35 people, including the mother and father, the two oldest children, both mothers-in-law, the pregnant girlfriend, the public health nurse, the teacher, the divorce court judge, two school nurses, the school attendance officer, and the juvenile worker. In an effort to interrupt the family pattern of blaming one another, each family member was asked to comment on what he or she thought the family problem really was. A "network effect" developed as people began to make serious positive suggestions as to how they could deal with some of the practical problems. The mother agreed to come to group therapy and to take classes in child rearing from a local teacher of special classes. The public health nurse undertook to make weekly visits to the mother, and the clinic nurse volunteered to have lunch with the mother weekly. The father agreed to attend Alcoholics Anonymous meetings. Latches were put on the doors so the 4-year-old could not get into his siblings' rooms to tear up their toys. A staff member functioning as a monitor was assigned to keep track of each person's contract.

The mother improved rapidly, and the children began doing better in school, although the parents did decide on a divorce. Difficulties continued relating to the issue of custody.

7

Case 6: Demons

Case 6 illustrates a problem in small rural communities, where fundamentalist and traditional cultural religious beliefs can influence how psychiatric problems present and are treated (Hoff 1990, 1992; Hoff and Galowa 1989; W. Hoff, G. Shapiro: "Traditional Healers and Community Health: A Review of the Literature Describing Projects Using Traditional Healers as Community Health Workers," Berkeley, CA, International Child Resource Institute, unpublished manuscript, 1990).

The director of a residential alcohol treatment program in a small rural town calls the psychiatrist, who is in a city about 3 hours away by plane. The director says:

"We have a 30-year-old woman here and she's really scared because demons are possessing her! She was drinking about 3 weeks ago but she's been sober since then so we don't think it's withdrawal or alcohol hallucinosis. She was fine last week, but now she feels that demons have taken total possession of her.

"They're talking to her about sexually oriented things, like rape, and she's been lying on the floor and holding the Bible between her legs to try to ward them off.

"We had her pastor come to visit her here at the program yesterday. He prayed over her, and she was better for about an hour after he left, but now she's a lot worse and feels the demons are taking over control completely.

"We don't know if we should keep having the pastor work with her, or ask you to prescribe medicine, or send her into the city to go to the psychiatric hospital. She comes from a small community of about

200 people that's 30 minutes away from here by plane. We've heard there's a lot of drinking and sexual abuse in her community—we're not sure if that could be related or not.

"A lot of people up here believe in demons, so we're not sure if it's a spiritual problem or a psychiatric problem. But it's getting to be too much for our staff to handle. We only have a 12-bed facility, and none of our staff has a lot of training in dual diagnosis. It's scaring some of the other patients. What would you recommend?"

On further questioning, the psychiatrist finds out that the woman has no known history of past treatment for mental problems. She has been a binge drinker at times in the past, but has not had heavy problem drinking compared with other people in her community and has no known alcohol-related medical problems or legal problems.

About 5 weeks ago, her 3-year-old daughter was shot in the chest accidentally by her 10-year-old nephew. She escorted the child on the plane ride into the city for surgical care. The daughter survived and now is doing well.

However, while she was in the city—a place she visits very infrequently—the woman started partying. She drank about three bottles of vodka over a weekend and also used marijuana. It is not clear if she used other drugs or engaged in any sexual activity.

On her way home to the village, the woman spent about a week in the town where the residential treatment center is, continuing to drink. Then she went into a mild withdrawal and went to the local hospital's emergency room, which led to her admission to the residential alcohol program. She has been there for 3 weeks and has done well until the last few days.

The psychiatrist telephones the pastor, who explains that he and many people in his congregation believe that spirits can come into a person and cause problems. He says that when he prayed with the woman the day before, she seemed to be getting better; he will be happy to visit and work with her again. However, when he talked to her, she mentioned some sexual matters, and he is worried that, under the influence of the demons, the woman will make sexual advances toward him. He also does not want to get into too close a relationship with the woman, because she might begin depending on him inappropriately. He feels she will do okay if he encourages her to pray more.

The psychiatrist agrees that the pastor should visit the patient again, because she seemed to get at least temporarily better after his last visit. The psychiatrist also phones the local general hospital to discuss with their physicians possible medications or hospitalization as a backup plan. (The local hospital is a small, 15-bed public general hospital staffed with four family physicians, some nurses, and a social worker, but familiarity with psychiatric diagnosis and medications is limited.)

Then the psychiatrist telephones the patient directly. He is uncomfortable about making recommendations at long distance for a patient he has never seen, but he is the nearest available psychiatrist. The patient agrees to talk to him and answers questions fairly well—except for occasional distractions when the demons are talking to her. She gives the following additional information.

She was married but has been separated for the past 7 years. She does not currently have a boyfriend but does have a number of other friends. Besides the daughter who was shot, she has another daughter, age 7, and two boys, one age 13 and one age 12. Both boys were "given away" to relatives to take care of.

She comes from a big family, with mother, father, six brothers, three sisters, and a number of more distant relatives. Some of them are "drinkers," but there is no family history of mental problems. She does not know of other people who have been possessed by demons.

She goes only rarely to a big city; on the recent visit, she blacked out and is very foggy on the sequence of events for the 4 days she was there.

At this point in the phone conversation, the woman stops talking to the psychiatrist for a short time. She says the voices are telling her they are going to rape her if she goes to sleep and are going to kill her. Then she returns to the conversation.

The psychiatrist feels her thinking is not that disorganized, except for this temporary lapse. There also does not appear to be a mood disorder that would meet the DSM-IV (American Psychiatric Association 1994) criteria. The woman does not remember taking other hallucinogens or substances besides alcohol and marijuana.

The psychiatrist asks about possible sexual activity, explaining that sometimes a combination of alcohol, marijuana, and sex might make a person more "sensitive" to the influences of demons, and that other women had reported being attacked sexually and then getting the demons. (In periodic field clinics in the rural town, the psychiatrist has come across nine other "demon" cases in the past 2 years, some of which presented this way.)

The woman seems very relieved to learn that this has happened to other people. She then reveals that when she returned from the big city to the rural town, she was drinking with a girlfriend and the girlfriend's husband. Her girlfriend "gets drunk real easy," and, while they were all drinking, the girlfriend made love to her husband right in front of her and then asked the patient to make love to her husband too. Over several days of drinking, she thinks she might have "given in" a couple of times but is not positive because she was "blacked out."

She noticed some pain in her rectum when she sobered up. She is afraid she was raped or had anal intercourse and might be torn or have an infection. She does not think they checked her very carefully at the hospital emergency room when she went in.

She says she feels better just from being able to talk this over with someone. The demons are not as loud now, and she thinks they might go away if she keeps up her prayers.

The psychiatrist encourages her to pray and to talk things over with the treatment center's staff. He talks again with the director who originally called, discussing a backup plan of medications and hospitalization in the event she does not improve. A physical examination by a female doctor is arranged to check on any damage to her anus that might need treatment and to discuss a possible human immunodeficiency virus (HIV) test. He also arranges for follow-up phone calls.

Differences in Health Beliefs

In remote rural settings, belief systems about health may be very different from what most psychiatrists are used to. Figure 7–1 is a tool designed to get at differences in health beliefs; along with a checklist of questions, it has been useful for teaching purposes (adapted from Kleinman 1980, 1987a, 1987b).

Figure 7–1 summarizes some key areas in which health beliefs are likely to differ, including 1) definition of the problem, 2) causal theories, 3) concepts of what the treatment should be and the role of the healer, 4) concepts about ideal states or desirable states of health, and 5) "rules of evidence" or what criteria or feedback is used to determine when the health state has been reached.

Table 7–1 gets at similar areas, including expectations and inner "mental models" about treatment, which can be important in dealing with the culturally different populations often found in remote rural areas.

In this case, the woman, as well as other people in her community, defines the problem as a spiritual one, caused by demons and requiring treatment that includes laying on of hands by an exorcist; use of Bibles and crosses to ward off the evil spirits; and a return by the woman to a life of aware spirituality, prayerfulness, and good deeds.

If this were an isolated case, it might not warrant extensive discus-

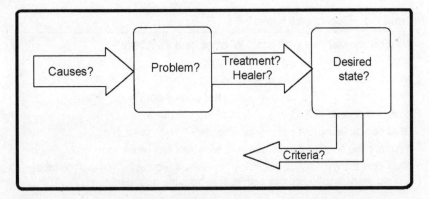

Figure 7–1. Gathering information to describe health beliefs. To find out about possible health beliefs, question patients as to 1) what they believe the problem or "diagnosis" is, 2) what their "causal theories" are, 3) what they believe "treatment" should consist of and expected role of "healer," 4) desired state when problem is gone or solved, and 5) how they will measure results or determine "treatment" has been successful.

sion. There are a number of "demon" cases in this region, however, and a variety of other similar types of cases occur elsewhere, especially in remote rural locations that have had little contact with the Western world until relatively recently.

Translation of Symptoms and Health Beliefs

A complex process appears to be at work in cases in which sometimes conflicting ideas and value systems interact; examples are Western disease classification versus indigenous ideas about illness, modern science versus folk culture, and biomedicine versus religious healing. The interaction can be considered "medical pluralism" and what Kleinman (1980, 1987a, 1987b) called "the shaping of symptoms."

In the past, "possession" cases in this region were considered "spirit intrusions," according to Eskimo religious beliefs. Treatment of such cases was left to spiritual healers or shamans, who performed rituals involving incantations and various physical measures. As missionaries came into the region, an overlay of fundamentalist Christian religious beliefs developed. Christian missionaries in some cases believed in laying on of hands and similar methods but thought shamans were "devil

Table 7–1.   Tool to elicit health beliefs

What do you call your problems? What name does it have?

What do you think caused your problem?

Why do you think it started when it did?

What does your sickness do to you? How does it work?

How severe is it? Will it have a short or long course?

What do you fear most about your disorder?

What are the chief problems that your sickness has caused for you?

What kind of treatment do you think you should receive? What are the most
   important results you hope to receive from the treatment?

Source.   Adapted from Kleinman 1980.

workers" and might even be the source of the affliction; this led to ambiguity concerning who had the power to exorcise spirits. Today there is another overlay of new beliefs; medical doctors, including psychiatrists, are more often in the region.

Psychiatrists tend to think in terms of a universal system of nosology such as DSM-IV. "Local" syndromes—which may be termed *culture-bound syndromes*—have been thought of as minor exceptions or possibly atypical cases within a "universal dominant" nosological system (Gaines 1979; Karp 1985; Prince and Tcheng-Laroche 1987). In this context, a comparison is usually made that says that disease X, occurring in society (or culture) A, is equivalent to disease Y in society (culture) B. In this kind of reclassification or translation, a possession case is "actually" schizophrenia or a hysterical reaction.

In this view, for something to be termed a *culture-bound syndrome*, it must be "untranslatable" by this process. In other words, it must be something that cannot be classified in Western psychiatric terms but absolutely requires examination of the cultural context in which it occurs. These untranslatable syndromes are amalgams embedded in the religious and cultural systems of their particular societies.

The translation process, however, may reflect a degree of ethnocentrism because the standard (culture or society B) is always a Western one. When certain phenomena embedded in a "local," "minor" cultural context are looked at from a "major," "dominant" point of view (i.e., a psychiatric viewpoint), there may be characteristics that do not fit the Western categories and that get left out of the translation. Kleinman (1987a, 1987b) called this a "category fallacy."

In this case, because a number of the people in the community believe in demons, possession has to be considered a shared experience. If this belief is to be translated as mental illness, there are a very large number of "patients"!

Varying Treatment Options

Treatment options in this case included an amalgam of traditional and religious healing on the one hand (Native elder who was also a lay minister in the church) and psychiatric treatment. If the society were not losing its traditional capacity to deal with this sort of case, the woman would probably never have become a possible candidate for psychiatric treatment. As the indigenous religious framework starts to change, the common cultural code or "social grammar" of disease breaks down. The psychiatric viewpoint often is brought in when the indigenous culture cannot deal with changing illness patterns within its own culture code. The indigenous view of illness then gets reshaped and translated into a "universal" system based on medical nosology (Eguchi 1991; Gaines 1979).

The traditional process can be represented as follows (Eguchi 1991):

personal suffering → religious suffering → possession → healing ritual (exorcism) → religious and communal stability.

This progression was rooted in the daily life of the village and was articulated as a religiously defined "set." It is now entangled with the psychiatric "set":

conflict → latent symptoms → acute symptoms → treatment and cessation of illness → individual understanding of or insight into the illness.

A new form of illness appears as a result of the interaction between traditional and modern values.

The psychiatrist who gets involved in these situations, trying to work as a translator across medical subcultures, is also subject to a process that Kleinman (1987a, 1987b) called "indigenization," as the "reality" of a medical specialist becomes entwined with and transformed by a powerful "popular reality." A two-way learning process is involved, not simply an attempt to fit a particular phenomenon into one set of criteria or another. When the psychiatrist attempts to appreciate fully the multi-faceted reality of the patient, who is caught between alternative categories or belief systems and does not fit well into any of them, the psychiatrist's own belief systems start to modify as a result of the communication process.

A villager struggling with a grief reaction put it this way:

> I used to believe in my traditional Native religion. There was a form of reincarnation so when a person died, their spirit came back. When the missionaries came, my beliefs had to change. Now it was "Heaven or Hell." But I didn't quite believe in these new ideas. Lately the missionaries' ideas are being questioned by all you psychiatrists, who see grief as a form of "depression." I can't deal with my grief the old way and don't really believe in reincarnation anymore, but I don't believe dead people just go to Hell either, which seems to be where the missionaries who came to my village thought all the Natives would end up. But "psychiatric insight" doesn't seem to help me deal with my grief either. So I'm lost—sort of like a "man without a country." What should I do?

After several experiences like this, the psychiatrist approaches the next patient a little bit less automatically.

The psychiatrist in this case did not employ a traditional Western approach. He contacted the local Native minister to get his views. He also contacted the local hospital but did not make an immediate referral into that system. The minister was encouraged to work further with the patient. When the psychiatrist talked with the patient, he referred to other "demon possession" situations, instead of immediately translating the woman's narrative into a DSM-III-R framework. In planning for aftercare in the village, he will probably seriously consider how the Native minister or traditional indigenous healers could collaborate. This would not have happened if the psychiatrist had not had repeated experiences of "indigenization," which made him more willing to rethink basic assumptions and appreciate how local people would perceive the situation.

Demons may not be found everywhere, but conflicting assumptions and values certainly are. Even business leaders are becoming aware of how their own assumptions can get in the way of both personal and organizational effectiveness. For example, Argyris (1982, 1985, 1990) trains executives to be more sensitive to "organizational defenses," such as telling the boss what you think he or she wants to hear and possibly covering up vital business information in the process. Argyris asks each trainee to recount a conflict with a client, colleague, or family member. The trainees have to recall not only what was said but what they were thinking and did *not* say. This develops awareness of the sweeping generalizations about others that determine what we say and do but that are never communicated. For example, a person might think, "Joe believes I'm incompetent," but never asks Joe directly about it; instead, he simply goes out of his way to make himself look competent to Joe.

The subtle patterns of reasoning that underlie behavior and perceptions, and that can block effective communication, need to be "surfaced" frequently in remote rural mental health work, often across a broad range of systems so that the practitioner can work successfully with teachers, police, tribal leaders, elders, and others.

The following is a general list of methods that have proven useful in these settings (Senge 1990a, 1990b). When advocating your view:

- Make your own reasoning explicit (i.e., say how you arrived at your view and the data on which it is based).
- Encourage others to explore your view (e.g., "Do you see gaps in my reasoning?").
- Encourage others to provide different views (i.e., "Do you have either different data or different conclusions, or both?").
- Actively inquire into others' views that differ from your own (i.e., "What are your views?" "How did you arrive at your view?" "Are you taking into account data that are different from what I have considered?").

When inquiring into others' views:

- State your assumptions clearly and acknowledge that they are assumptions if you are making assumptions about others' views.
- State the "data" on which your assumptions are based.
- Do not bother asking questions if you are not genuinely interested in the others' response (i.e., if you are only trying to be polite or to show the others up).

When you arrive at an impasse (others no longer appear open to inquiring into their own views):

- Ask what data or logic might change their views.
- Ask if there is any way you might together design an experiment (or some other inquiry) that might provide new information.

When you or others are hesitant to express your views or to experiment with alternative ideas:

- Encourage them (or you) to think out loud about what might be making it difficult (i.e., "What is it about this situation, and about me or others, that is making open exchange difficult?").
- Design with others ways of overcoming these barriers if there is mutual desire to do so.

The point is not to follow such guidelines slavishly but to use them to keep in mind the spirit of balancing inquiry and advocacy. Like any "formula" for starting on one of the learning disciplines, they should be used as "training wheels" on your first bicycle. They help to get you started and give you a feel for what it is like to "ride," to practice inquiry with advocacy. As you gain skill, they can and probably should be discarded. It is helpful to come back to them periodically, however, when you encounter some rough terrain.

Another useful list of questions has been developed at the Marriage and Family Therapy Clinic at the University of Iowa (Fleuridas et al. 1986). These build on concepts such as "circular questioning," "neutrality," and "hypothesizing." The neutral stance means not making taken-for-granted assumptions about families. Instead, hypotheses are made and revised as new evidence comes to light. A special type of questioning is used to check out the hypotheses; information is solicited from the family members regarding their opinion and experience of 1) the family's presenting concern; 2) sequences of interactions, usually related to the problem; and 3) differences in their relationships over time.

The idea of "circularity" emphasizes cyclical sequences of interactions that interconnect with family beliefs. These patterns of relating may serve to perpetuate dysfunctional behaviors and cognitions. Individuals are best understood within their interrelational contexts. A comprehensive, systemic view of the family focuses on the evolving relationships of the family members within their environmental, historical, developmental, and ideological contexts.

Who "Owns" the Problem?

As in other cases in this book, this case has a number of potential "owners." One key dilemma for the psychiatrist is how much to involve Native healers or fundamentalist ministers and how much to rely only on health professionals.

From the patient's point of view, and from that of others in her community, demons are not hallucinations but are real, and a treatment involving laying on of hands, and possible exorcism, might be preferred. From the health system's point of view, the patient has a medical-psychiatric condition and would benefit from professional help.

In this case, the psychiatrist attempted to straddle the fence by both arranging for medical care and involving a local minister. It is not always possible to do this. Some traditional treatments may be seen as dangerous by the medical profession, although local people believe in them. Other difficulties may arise if the Native healer wants to use unorthodox methods in a treatment facility that has rules about licensing, privileging, and accreditation.

Because small communities are sensitive to the nuances of outsiders' ideas and actions, the psychiatrist working in these situations needs to be well tuned in so as to avoid getting caught up in factionalism or inadvertently offending a sizable chunk of the community.

Although separation of church and state is attempted, fundamentalist ministers have been hired in some remote rural locations as alcohol counselors or in similar government-funded jobs. When there is more than one fundamentalist religious group in the community, each with strong views, deep divisions and conflicts within the community can occur. For example, the psychiatrist may be asked to help deal with a family problem and then discover that some members of the family belong to one church, others have been converted to a rival church, and one of the pastors is also the local counselor!

What Can Be Done for the Immediate Problem?

The psychiatrist in this case considered various medical and psychiatric conditions that might present the way this patient did, including the possibility of a delayed drug withdrawal reaction. For example, the patient might have taken long-acting benzodiazepines for an extended period of time while "partying," although the lapse of 3 weeks seemed too long unless the history was wrong and she had not really been "detoxed" for that whole period. Or people in the residential facility might have had access to drugs while in the program. However, the most likely diagnosis, at least from a standard psychiatric perspective, seemed to be a form of post-rape trauma syndrome, expressing itself in the form it did because of the woman's strong religious convictions.

The psychiatrist discussed the physical examination and laboratory test results with the psychiatric nurse at the regional general hospital and concluded that there was no hard evidence of medical problems, including withdrawal, that would account for the presenting symptoms. He talked by phone again with the staff at the residential alcohol facility and worked out a plan whereby the psychiatric nurse would see the patient for further supportive counseling, and the alcohol treatment staff would talk with her about substance abuse problems.

The minister was encouraged to continue his visits. The woman reportedly improved rapidly and then returned to the village. The regional mental health and alcohol staff discussed the situation with the village paraprofessional health worker, who will be on the lookout for early warning signs of difficulties and will call the backup social worker or family physician as needed. The Native minister in the town made contact with the village minister so that additional supportive counseling could be provided. Because of some friction between the village minister and the indigenous healers in the village, it was decided not to make active attempts to involve traditional healers for the time being.

One issue that sometimes comes up in cases like this is how best to involve the local doctors. The alcohol program director originally called the psychiatrist, not the local hospital doctors. If the psychiatrist allows this bypass to continue, the local doctors will learn nothing, needed medical checks will not take place, and more cases that could be handled locally will come to the psychiatrist in the future. If all the consultation is routed through the local doctors, however, it is unlikely the case will be handled well for reasons similar to those discussed in Case 3 (Chapter 4)—too many constraints on local staff so that only quick fixes tend to be done.

The approach used by the psychiatrist in this case was aimed at getting everyone involved to the degree possible. He took on something of a "translator" or "culture-broker" role, working with local groups who had different beliefs about the causes of the problem and what should be done.

What Else Could Be Done?

A number of remote rural communities in Alaska are trying to revive some of the traditional cultural ceremonies. Other communities, feeling they have lost touch with their cultural roots, have invited medicine men and elders from Canada or other parts of the United States to help them rebuild traditions and ceremonies. "Healing Gatherings," as well as a form of traditional group therapy known as the "Talking Circle," are being used. A few communities have tried to involve church groups through such activities as "Sacred Circles" (like "Talking Circles" with religious symbolism amplified), Alcoholics Victorious (similar to Alcoholics Anonymous but with Bible study added), and so on.

A "Traditional Healing Project" has been in operation for some time in one region of the state; local mental health staff can systematically assemble and read literature about traditional practices and folk medicine and talk with elders who serve as cultural mentors to the program. This project includes looking at the intake process for Yupik psychiatric patients. Interviews are done in the Yupik language and then in English with the same patient through a translator. The types of information obtained, and the types of treatment plans, are then compared in great detail.

In at least one region, local indigenous healers have held "traditional medicine" workshops to exchange information about their methods. Attempts have been made in some regions to collect information from elders about herbal treatments, midwives' practices, and various folk medicine remedies. Because of the legacy of missionaries who convinced many that traditional dances, ceremonies, and other practices were evil and should be suppressed, as well as the ambivalence of some Native people who want to "modernize," it is difficult to find out as much as might be desirable about local ethnopsychology (Craig 1988; Flanders 1991; McNabb 1991; Van Stone 1964).

One region has identified its traditional healers and is holding "tribal doctors" workshops to plan future projects to help Native youth, as well as to demonstrate traditional healing practices and make careful descriptions of various aspects, terms, and concepts that are involved. There is also interest in how the tribal doctors and the primary health care system could begin to work more cooperatively with each other (Fortuine 1988, 1989, 1993; Hoff 1990, 1992; Hoff and Shapiro, unpublished manuscript, 1990; Streather 1991; Tan et al. 1988).

Obstacles to many of these efforts are the disincentives built into the current health system for involving indigenous healers. If a villager wants to see a psychiatrist, air travel costs from the village to the clinic in the regional hub town are reimbursable by Medicaid. If the same patient wants to fly to another village to see an indigenous healer, the costs would not be reimbursable. Licensing and privileging of indigenous healers, so they can see people in hospital facilities, is also a problem. Unfortunately, many other policies and procedures also work to discourage collaborative efforts between psychiatrists and indigenous healers.

What Should the Psychiatrist's Role Be?

Sometimes the religious and the psychiatric systems, or the indigenous and the psychiatric systems, operate completely autonomously with no cross-connections. The amount of cooperation is largely a function of how interested the psychiatrist is in contacting and communicating with these other systems. It is rare for religious and indigenous healers to make the first move to involve psychiatrists.

In a few places, attempts at cooperation are made, as in this case, with some cross-referral of patients. Psychiatrists in some cases have been able to observe local healers at work and to try to learn some of their approaches. A health careers program in the state is designed to encourage Native high school students to consider careers in health-related fields. One student who was interested in psychiatry took a summer enrichment program in which she studied part-time with local and indigenous healers and part-time with a psychiatrist to try to learn biculturally.

Real collaboration between leaders or indigenous healers and mental health staff is possible. In projects that involve elders and scientists as equal partners in research activities, the psychiatrist's role is to help train Native interviewers so that, when traditional practices are demonstrated and described, full and "rich" descriptions of the psychological aspects are possible. Representatives from the World Health Organization's Expert Committee on Traditional Healing are also involved with these projects.

There are numerous other opportunities for traditional healers or religious leaders and psychiatrists to work together and learn from each other—for example, solving some of the problems of lack of specialized foster care for disabled patients by helping church groups set up volunteer homes, and organizing pastoral counseling training programs for village counselors.

Another Point of View

Like the others in this book, the case of the woman possessed by demons can be viewed from different perspectives, depending on cultural background and life experience. The following comments by an Iñupiaq Eskimo cultural mentor give a picture of how local people might perceive the issues. This is of course only one person's opinion; however, in our experience, these comments are fairly typical in this region.

An Iñupiaq View of the Problem

In this case, we are dealing with taboos, evil or evil spirits, and the role of medicine men and medicine women. A basic principle is that when a force gets hidden, it gets stronger and stronger and eventually becomes uncontrollable.

We have terms in Eskimo describing the "world of hard work and communications" and the "world of leisure and pleasure." This pleasure world is associated with not being conscious. When you are not conscious, evil powers tend to sprout up. Communication and discipline are needed to keep the evil powers from getting stronger. Spirituality has to be "awake." What is needed is prayerfulness and good deeds.

We feel that evil spirits eat off a person's brain. A person can then become paranoid, selfish, abusive, unhuman-like, with misuse of his or her power exhibiting instead the chaotic power of evil that is out of hand.

A medicine person can develop a power base and can use it to create mystical things. That person needs to be prayerful and fear God, however. If the person is weak as far as discipline, the false god of pleasure and leisure can take over.

In this case, the woman was not doing hard work and practicing discipline. Instead, she became helpless and consumed by an evil power—all her mind and body. Treatment in this case would be to call one of our Native ministers for a laying on of hands. The woman needs a casting out of the evil powers, so she can change and be mindful of God and the power of prayer. She has to want to change—she will have to be strong, have faith and belief, and cooperate with the healers.

Traditionally there are angels of the North, South, East, and West—powerful forces that serve as wardens and guardians, watching over us until we are conscious and able to think for ourselves. Our forefathers and grandparents were strong believers in the work of God. There were taboos connected with "snares," "traps," and "fishnets," and we always had to rest on Sundays.

In this woman's case, however, there is a lack of being spiritual or disciplined. She really needs to ask from her heart for God to help her.

If she is admitted to the local alcohol program, a spiritual mentor needs to be found for her. Crosses could be put in her room in each of "the Four Directions"—North, South, East, and West. She could put another cross on.

She has to want to be spiritual, to convert leisure into work, and pleasure into discipline. She has to make her choice. Like many people—especially the young people and the suicides—the enemy is trying to get to her. She should be given a Bible and told to go to church.

We have many stories up here as well as personal experiences with powerful forces. For example, a force that seems to be stronger with men might just lift your bed suddenly up. Or a man living alone, whose house is usually a mess, might notice that this time the house is nice and clean, with a big white dog lying on his bed, and then when he comes back again the house is messy and the dog is gone.

There are stories of a time when the bar was open here, and a man with a long white robe walked in. He had hooves instead of shoes. He suddenly disappeared. Forty children at the recreation center saw this same man, dressed in white with hooves instead of feet, and all ran outside very scared.

In the Arctic, evil forces may be stronger because we had more shamans and medicine people. Only three to four generations ago we were still having ritualistic ceremonies.

The trail between here and a nearby village, for example, has lights off in the distance; when you are riding on that trail by snow machine or by sled dog, you have to be careful not to go off and follow those lights in the dark or you will get lost. The shelter cabins along this trail are often haunted as well.

Before the missionaries came, we had strong taboos. Children were obedient to their parents. There was no radio, no television, no basketball, but we were God fearing. When the missionaries "hit the beach," our taboos were lifted. The evil powers started to get stronger. God is strong all the time, but the people are being attacked more.

Five generations ago, we had strong beliefs, loved each other, and cared for each other. Now the people are weakened. There is defiance against the church and the government, so there is nothing to stand on. They added too many rules when they brought the church up here. They suppressed our language, dances, and songs. Now our leaders pray for us, but we really do not know what our beliefs are anymore.

The psychiatrist's role in this type of case should be to refer the patient to the Native minister for the exorcism and spiritual healing that are needed. The problem is not a psychiatric problem—it is a spiritual one.

Examples From Other Settings

In various parts of the world, the primary health care system and traditional healers are encouraged to work together. In a project in Ghana, healers were taught preventative and promotive measures, family planning, the use of allopathic medicines, and basic first aid. In Nepal, traditional practitioners learned how to recognize and manage tuberculosis and leprosy. In Brazil, local healers were trained to integrate oral rehydration therapy with their own indigenous practices aimed at achieving child survival. Because many traditional healers conceptualize their work as an integrated system to heal body, mind, and spirit, even programs that appear to concern physical health have many mental health aspects.

Training Traditional Healers in Swaziland

The Kingdom of Swaziland is one of the smallest countries in Africa (Hoff 1990, 1992; Hoff and Shapiro, unpublished manuscript, 1990). It has an estimated population of 721,000 and is approximately equivalent in size to the state of Rhode Island. Although it has a fairly well-developed system of health services for its size, it still has high rates of infant, child, and maternal mortality. Infant mortality, for example, is more than

150 per 1,000 live births. There are few villages, and most families live apart from each other in rural homesteads. This scattered and independent pattern of living renders the provision of health services particularly difficult.

Traditional healing in Swaziland, as in most African countries, is a long-established and widely accepted indigenous health system. It is estimated that there are between 5,000 and 8,000 traditional healers who actively practice as herbalists, midwives, spirit mediums, and faith healers. The ratio of healers to patients is approximately 1 to 100, whereas the ratio of modern trained doctors is only about 1 to 7,000. The vast majority of healers live in rural areas; most modern doctors practice in towns or cities. It is common for healers to go to the family homestead to diagnose and treat a sick patient; modern doctors rarely do this.

Although most Swazis do use the services of local clinics and hospitals, approximately 85% of the population still seek the help of traditional healers for many conditions. Public health experts have therefore looked for ways to build on the traditional system, hoping to improve access to care for the rural people and to improve infant mortality.

Healers in Swaziland often give a traditional type of "vaccination" to protect the body from certain illnesses or to ward off evil spirits. They make small cuts in the skin with a knife or razor blade and then rub in a specific herbal mixture to impregnate the superficial skin layer with the protective herbs. Although many Swazis believe that these vaccinations are helpful, there is as yet no scientific evidence to indicate how effective they are. However, health authorities do not believe they cause serious harm, provided that clean instruments are used.

Public health experts have built on this practice by explaining that modern immunizations are similar to traditional practices and that substances can be injected into the skin to protect a child from modern diseases. Nurses were willing to accept traditional immunizations if performed under hygienic conditions, and they encouraged healers to refer patients to the clinics to obtain modern immunizations as well. Some nurses suggested to the healers in their communities that traditional immunizations would protect half the child and modern immunizations would protect the other half.

This view of immunization was more readily understood by the healers, and they began to be open to the idea of cooperating with the nurses to protect children from diseases. Evaluation data showed evidence that healers began referring children to clinics for checkups and immunizations.

Cultures Clash in Kake

Events in an Alaskan community demonstrate what can happen when cultures are at odds at the local level. Psychiatrists need to be aware of how strong such feelings can be, because mental health efforts to promote cultural pride and identity or to learn from and work with traditional healers may inadvertently trigger conflict.

Kake is a town of 750 that sprawls along the northwest shore of an island in southeast Alaska. The Tlingit people who live there have a stormy history of contact with the white culture, including battles with explorers and traders; in 1869, the United States Army shelled and destroyed the village after villagers killed two traders in revenge for the shooting of a Native.

After missionaries came to the island and a school was established, village leaders held a formal ceremony in 1912 to celebrate the end of the old traditions and the advent of a new culture. A silver spike, the symbol of "our complete change in beliefs," was driven into the newly constructed wooden main street. Shortly thereafter, villagers cut down and burned the totem poles that stood next to their homes and hid or destroyed their traditional ceremonial regalia.

In recent years, the community has been deeply divided about traditional cultural activities. Some feel that practices like traditional ceremonial dancing and totem carving are evil, that some of the masks represent demonic powers, and that the regalia is like the idols the Bible warns against. Others are very concerned about the youth in the community, who seem to lack knowledge of who they are, drink heavily, and are often suicidal. This group has been trying to promote a cultural revival, teaching dance, regalia making, Tlingit language, and mask carving in the local school and in after-school programs.

A Pentecostal minister, herself a Tlingit, recently came to Kake and preached at a church service that totems, clan hats, and other Native art are demonic and that Native dancing is akin to worshiping Satan. Several nights after she preached, a group of village teenagers tossed rock-and-roll tapes, heavy metal T-shirts, and bottles of alcohol into a flaming 50-gallon barrel. Among the ashes, the town's fire chief also found remnants of what appeared to be traditional artwork and dance regalia. A dozen or so troubled teenagers were "saved" at the revival, according to many who attended, and the fire was a way to purge old devils.

Townspeople are now quite upset. The controversy has struck at the heart of Kake's sense of identity, dividing friends and family who no longer speak to one another. "It's our history repeating itself," said one of the cultural revival leaders when she heard she had been called evil and a devil worshiper, "but this time it's our own people."

Mental Health Care in Rural India

The study summarized here (Kapur 1975) is one of the few that deals with an important aspect of mental health care in rural areas: utilization of services and survey methods that could be used to establish the need for additional work with traditional practitioners. The study of mental health care in rural areas focused on the conceptual frameworks of various traditional and modern healers. An attitude survey asked about the type of healer favored by the local residents for psychiatric consultation; then a survey of those with symptoms was carried out to learn whom they had actually consulted.

Basic questions were:

- What are the cultural anticipations and stereotypes about basic health workers compared with traditional healers?
- What agencies are available in the villages for helping mentally ill persons?
- What are the conceptual frameworks within which these agencies operate?
- How important are these conceptual frameworks to the potential clients?
- Do the villagers consult at all when in psychological distress?
- What factors promote or hinder such consultation?
- Whom do people prefer to consult when they have psychiatric symptoms: traditional healers or modern practitioners? What factors dictate the preference?
- How do people view the primary health centers and the basic health workers? What potential do these centers have for taking up the responsibility for mental health care?

The results of the study showed that 32% of the men and 40% of the women had one or more psychiatric symptoms. "Possession" cases consulted least with any type of practitioner. Those with more psychiatric symptoms tended to get more consultation. The majority (48%) of those surveyed had consulted with both modern and traditional healers; 23% of the men and 10% of the women had consulted only a traditional healer; 30% of the men and 42% of the women had consulted a doctor and had not consulted a traditional healer. There were no differences by age, education, or income categories. It was not true that villagers did not consult when in psychiatric distress: 59% of those with symptoms had consulted, with 24% having consulted recently, in the month before the survey.

Of the total sample of 1,233, 9% had consulted some type of healer for psychiatric symptoms in the past month. All of the epileptic and psychotic persons in need of attention appeared to have consulted someone. Modern doctors were the preferred source of help; claims that villagers generally go to traditional healers first for psychiatric problems were not validated, except for cases of possession symptoms, of whom hardly anyone preferred the modern doctor, and psychotic patients, of whom about 50% had consulted a traditional healer only.

There is an extreme shortage of psychiatrists, and any increase in professionally trained staff is expected to be absorbed immediately by the big cities. Therefore, alternative methods of delivering services are needed for rural areas. Innovative mental health programs may rely 1) on semiprofessionals and nonprofessionals, with short periods of training; 2) on use of primary health centers, with general doctors, a team of nurses, plus basic health workers and family planning workers; and 3) on professionals for backup at the district level.

8

Case 7: How About Strip Searches?

This case illustrates legal issues that may come up when efforts to decrease alcohol abuse in remote rural communities are made (Murray and Kupinsky 1982; O'Neil 1986; Samson 1992; Sandler and Lakey 1982; Santos et al. 1993; Whyte 1982). Many psychiatrists must now contend with legal and ethical issues impacting on their practice; managed care, malpractice problems, and treatment guidelines are increasing concerns. In the case presented in this chapter, some of the remote rural variations on these issues are raised.

In a small fishing village about 100 miles away from the nearest small town, a drunken youth fell into the river and drowned. That tragedy led the village council to start searching all visitors. Although the term *strip searches* was used, it was not clear whether this was just a pat-down or whether people might on occasion have to remove their clothes completely. Also, the exact nature of the searches (e.g., whether women would be assigned to search women and men to search men) was not clearly spelled out. In addition, the council gave village police authority to search the homes of those suspected of drinking.

The village council wanted the flow of bootleg liquor into the community to stop and did not see any way to do this without the search policy. "We don't want alcohol to poison our community," the council administrator said.

The state government, however, put the village council on notice that the mandatory searches for drugs and alcohol were illegal. State workers who needed to visit the village protested the searches, claiming their constitutional rights against unreasonable search were being violated. In response, state officials told workers not to go to the village while the searches continue. Employees of the school district, the public health nursing office, the Department of Family and Youth Services, and the utilities company were given the option by their employers not to travel to the village.

The state proposed various measures to resolve the problem, including issuing identification cards for state employees to show to village residents on request; the state workers would also state the nature of their business in the village. State officials further suggested that the villagers hold a vote to ban possession of alcohol in their village. This can be done under a state "local option" law that gives each village "local control" over its alcohol policies. At present, the village bans importation of alcohol but not possession. Finally, the state suggested that villagers could conduct voluntary searches and then secure search warrants when there is probable cause to believe any baggage contains alcohol.

This remote village feels that state law enforcement is slow to respond when they call for help. The village is too small to have its own state trooper—the nearest is about an hour away by plane, when weather permits flights. The village council has therefore exerted local control to prevent more alcohol-related deaths in its community. Council members want to solve their own problems in their own way rather than relying on a distant state bureaucracy.

From a psychiatric point of view, there are numerous alcohol-related health and mental health problems in this community. If the local people could sober up, a considerable reduction in associated psychiatric problems could be expected.

Cultural factors are at work here too. The fishing village consists of members of an Eskimo group that considers it has "tribal sovereignty." Although the village is in the United States, villagers do not especially identify as United States citizens, pointing out that their ancestors were on the land thousands of years before the United States government with its laws and constitutional rights was established. Under the tribal sovereignty principle, some neighboring villages are setting up tribal courts that will operate under their own tribal laws.

Local Control Versus Central Standardization

Statewide groups, wanting to develop laws, programs, and approaches to public policy issues that will apply across the board and will be fair to everyone, often find themselves at odds with local communities whose unique problems do not fit the general solutions. There are issues here of centralization versus decentralization and local control; to what extent legal systems should be used to control people's behavior; and, in this case, whose legal system should be considered primary. Psychiatrists who are now debating the use of national practice guidelines have raised questions about how to address regional diversity and are worried about "one-size-fits-all" or cookbook approaches.

Many variations on this "central standardization versus local control" theme arise in remote rural psychiatric work in Alaska. The villagers in this case, for example, feel they do not fit into the statewide laws and regulations.

Some incidents have a direct impact on clinical care. A rural judge heard a case in which it seemed clear to the mental health team that child abuse was taking place in the home. The judge, sensitive to local concerns about removing children from the home, instead gave a court order to the parent that no child abuse take place and that certain parental behaviors take place. If there was no compliance, the child could then be removed. The mental health team felt that the judge was exposing the child to unnecessary risk of additional abuse by trying to legislate good parental behavior in this way.

Other cases may seem removed from clinical concerns at first but may indirectly affect people's perceptions of their identity. This applies to fish and game regulations that are strongly supported by commercial and sports groups who want access to rural fishing on a "fair" basis and are opposed by locals who want protection for their unique subsistence lifestyle. It applies to oil and mineral rights when regional and statewide groups with "subsurface" rights want to develop oil and mineral rights, locals want to hunt and fish on the surface of that same land, and environmentalists are concerned about pollution and interference with animal migration patterns. It applies to many other issues of local versus central control, including numerous health issues. These range from hiring standards, and which rules for staff qualifications should be used (local people with experience versus outsiders with professional degrees), to how child protection cases should be handled (villages that want to handle them inside the group versus state reporting requirements), to facility licensing questions (Natives' desire for programs in natural, camplike wilderness settings versus requirements for sprinkler systems and other safety measures to meet state regulations or codes). There may even be questions about whether Native foods such as seal meat are sanitary and can be served in accredited hospitals to patients who are not used to standard hospital food.

Psychiatrists may be drawn into the resulting battles in a variety of ways. They may serve on teams carrying out psychosocial "impact studies" or testify at hearings on these issues. For example, at the time of the installation of the Alaska pipeline, and again at the time of the Exxon Valdez oil spill, psychiatrists were asked to participate in multidisciplinary teams of social scientists attempting to assess the human impacts of these events.

Psychiatrists and other mental health professionals may get involved in trying to help local programs meet national and state program standards. For example, a central headquarters will decide that a new management information system needs to be put into place and that the rural alcohol or mental health programs need to comply with various report requirements. The local people may feel these requirements are burdensome and do not make sense for their counselors, some of whom may have difficulty speaking English and even more difficulty filling out complicated computer database forms. They may request help from local psychiatrists to fight what they consider the unrealistic demands of distant bureaucracies.

An additional concern here is the impact on mental health in local communities that have repeatedly battled statewide interests, on multiple fronts, and lost. Remote rural communities often feel that too many key decisions are made by powerful outside interests. Feelings of powerlessness, due to the external locus of control, and a degree of learned helplessness can result. Communities may ask psychiatrists to support their efforts at "empowerment" to deal with these concerns and may see this as definitely a mental health issue.

The "local option" law was an attempt by the state of Alaska to allow local communities to decide how to handle control of alcohol, within an overall state framework. This law permits communities to prohibit or restrict the sale of alcoholic beverages if they vote to do so. Because people may purchase alcohol in other locations that do not have the prohibition and then get it shipped in, or claim that the alcohol is just for their "personal use" rather than for sale, the law limits the quantities that may be imported or deemed to be for personal use. Local communities have further options under this law to adopt ordinances restricting importation and possession or consumption of alcoholic beverages. As this case shows, however, there are many "gray-zone" questions left unanswered by this approach.

Psychiatrists involved in backup roles with small rural communities are apt to encounter variations on this general problem. Local communities may want waivers on licensing requirements for staff, because locals do not have the professional qualifications, and outsiders who are qualified usually do not stay long in the community or understand local issues very well. There may be debates about the types of services that are offered—for example, to what degree folk medicine practices by local healers should be encouraged, sanctioned, and funded.

An example of the often unexpected ways this conflict can surface occurred when a psychiatrist went to a small remote community where a town meeting had been scheduled. He was told there had been some recent deaths in the village, and the local people wanted to talk over their feelings. The psychiatrist went to the meeting expecting people to talk about their grief.

These feelings were in fact present, but the main issue people wanted to talk about was the legal requirement for autopsies after certain types of alcohol-related and violent deaths. Because the village had no coroner, the bodies had to be sent to the regional hub town. There was often some delay before the body was returned for the funeral, and villagers felt that the bodies were frequently not in the best condition when they came back. Moreover, because of other regulations, bills for the transportation costs associated with sending the body for autopsy were being sent to relatives of the deceased.

What the psychiatrist had expected to be a group meeting about grief became largely a discussion of what villagers might do politically and legally to gain more local control over how autopsies were handled. His role was to help local tribal leaders get legal consultation on the laws and regulations governing autopsies, so that they could help the villagers identify possible intervention points.

Who "Owns" the Problem?

It is still unclear in this and similar cases how much "tribal rights" can be exercised, especially when they are in conflict with the United States Constitution. Many American Indian and Alaska Native tribes consider they have "sovereign nation" status and should be negotiated with independently, as a foreign government would be.

Federal laws now encourage attempts by American Indians and Alaska Natives to move toward self-determination and self-governance. Local tribal courts, as mentioned above, which follow locally developed

laws and enforcement strategies, are widespread in many American Indian communities and are beginning in some Alaska Native villages.
Whole hospital systems, including the psychiatry departments, are being contracted out by the federal government to tribal groups under the
self-determination and self-governance philosophy. The psychiatrist
working with these programs may find that virtually every aspect of
practice is considered a local control issue. Abortion policies, adoption
policies, recruiting of staff, state and federal standards, reporting requirements for problems like child abuse, and multiple other issues may
be viewed by tribal groups as potentially contestable legally or as take-
over targets so that there can be more local community input.

Taking child abuse as an example, there are local efforts by many
Alaska Native villages to use "Talking Circles," a form of group discussion and therapy in which what is said in the group is supposed to stay
in the group and remain confidential. When topics such as child abuse
or child sexual abuse come up, activities may be described that are re-
portable under state reporting statutes. Group members, however, may
feel strongly that they should handle the problem in their own way and
may refuse to report to state authorities. Professional staff involved with
child protection efforts are usually opposed to violations of the reporting
statutes, and extremely polarized situations can result.

In other cases, treatment camps in wilderness settings may have difficulty complying with treatment-facility codes regarding fire safety,
sprinkler systems, barrier-free access for people with disabilities, and so
on. Patient safety regulations may have some special twists—for example, figuring out how best to protect residents at a wilderness camp from
bears and how much to spend on safety precautions. In some of these
situations, there are no easy answers as to where to draw the line, or who
gets to decide, on the ownership issue.

What Can Be Done for the Immediate Problem?

In this case, the community stuck to its position while awaiting further
legal tests. Local village leaders reported, "When we first started the
searches, they [persons and organizations affected] let us know they
thought it was illegal. . . . But we were never afraid because we were ex-
ercising our rights as a tribal government to make our own laws for the
community." The tribal government did not tolerate alcohol in the vil-

lage; on the third offense, the offender received a ticket to another village and was not allowed to return.

Other villages formed tribal government systems that have enacted similar measures to combat the availability of alcohol. Alcohol-related crimes such as wife beating, child molestation, stabbing, and assault have been almost nonexistent since the villagers started searching new arrivals. Problems that have been going on for "years and years and years" were now being solved.

There were still some problems with the search-and-seizure effort. Law enforcement personnel employed by the traditional government were not allowed to conduct searches on children, some of whom are used to bring in drugs. Another problem is that winter opened up travel by snow machine between villages, which allowed alcohol and marijuana to be transported.

Law enforcement officials applauded the efforts of the villagers, although they could officially condone what is possibly an unconstitutional way to deal with the problem of illicit drugs and alcohol. From a health and mental health standpoint, the villagers' approach seemed to be working, although it was still in conflict with the United States Constitution.

What Else Could Be Done?

Other remote rural communities are watching what happens in this case with considerable interest to see if they might be able to use a similar approach. Self-government and increased tribal sovereignty are being negotiated wherever possible. This has been happening relatively rapidly so that soon all the Indian Health Service federal programs in Alaska, for example, may be contracted out to tribes to operate themselves. Until 1971, the programs, including hospitals, clinics, and village programs throughout Alaska, were all operated directly by the federal government.

The tendency for small communities to want to be more autonomous and run their own affairs is desirable in that it is generally associated with improved attitudes about being in control, being responsible, and having more sense of community spirit and identity. There are trade-offs, however. For example, economies of scale possible with centralized programming are reduced. In addition, program monitoring and technical assistance efforts are made more difficult when everyone wants to "do their own thing."

What Should the Psychiatrist's Role Be?

True empowerment of local communities involves more than just giving local people money and letting them run their own programs. Because there is a lack of local economic base in most of these remote rural communities, the money tends to come from outside. Locals want to "cut the apron strings" of dependency and paternalism but seldom want to "cut the purse strings" of state and federal funding. A sort of angry, ambivalent dependency results.

Psychiatrists can help in training and educational efforts with local people to improve their abilities at problem solving, communications, and group dynamics. They can also play an interface or "culture-broker" role, using a form of shuttle diplomacy between remote rural communities and larger centralized policy-making groups. Their attempt is to help negotiate "all-win" solutions and to prevent the escalation process that usually leads to the eventual squashing of local interests.

Empowerment is a buzzword in rural Alaska. When it is really discussed, it is apparent that it is a rubber-band concept that can be stretched different ways by different people to mean different things. Psychiatrists need to think critically about this concept, because they will probably be asked to do all sorts of things based on empowerment as a rationale promoted by locals.

To move beyond involvement and truly empower means to look at relationships. If one group is going to do something to empower another group, the one doing the empowering implicitly believes that the other people are weak and need to be made whole. The group to be empowered is still dependent on the one doing the empowering.

For real empowerment, issues such as reciprocity, problem-solving skills, communication, and group dynamics and concerns about money, power, ego, and control need to be addressed. A systemic view, longer-term thinking, involvement of multiple levels in a problem-solving effort, and avoidance of prepackaged programs and quick fixes are often needed. It is also clear that, in many communities, not everyone wants to be empowered, raising questions about who speaks for the community when self-determination is being promoted.

Another Point of View

On issues like the ones in this case, because local people may see things rather differently from the professionals, it can be helpful to talk directly to key informants and then compare with professional points of view. The local people may not describe events in terms a psychiatrist is used to, but this in itself can be quite informative. If there is going to be an attempt at intervention, whether it be shuttle diplomacy, public health education and social marketing, or some other approach, it can be very important first to hear all the different points of view.

An account of the search case was read to an Alaska Native who felt comfortable with the interviewer; her comments were written down verbatim. This demonstrates which ideas tend to be associated, perhaps in quite different ways from a psychiatrist's conceptualization. For example, the comments jump from the strip search case to control of decision making of all types, including decisions about the school system. Such revelations of the inner logic used by the informant and other local people, and of how information is categorized, may be essential to understand before trying to be of help. Possible stereotypes, local terms and concepts, unwarranted generalizations, and misunderstandings that might need to be addressed by a mediator trying to find some common ground and negotiate a solution between the polarized factions in this case need to be identified as part of the diagnostic workup of the conflict situation.

An Alaska Native's View of the Problem

In this case, the state public health nurse should be fired! She is not serving the village. She's not helping. She should be the last one trying to stop the searches.

The village should be more self-sufficient. They need more local control of schools and more local control of all decision making.

The state is being genocidal and is against self-determination. The local people should be making their own decisions about their own health. The state is finding every reason in the book to stop local decisions. The state says "local option" but doesn't really mean it. In former times, we had strong village councils. Now it's usurped by the state, the federal government, and the courts, all fragmenting the village decision-making process.

Once a village makes a decision, we should support it. We have a number of terms in Eskimo dealing with these ideas. There is a word for village decision making, which is the same term we use for Christ. There is another term for "speaking with one mind."

Traditionally, villagers would get together and form a circle to talk over important issues. Each person had a voice. When the position was unanimous, very strong decisions could be reached and enforced. There might be very strict curfews, for example. There would be no policemen, but lots of power held by the village council. If there were enough violations, a family could even be "blue ticketed" out of town.

There was no stealing. No one ever locked up their cabins or homes. People did make little marks on personal belongings so they could identify them. People were honest, and it was a safe place to live. There was little alcohol use until contact with the whalers, who taught us how to distill hard liquor.

Nowadays our tribal laws are not effective at the village level. The courts try to talk for us. It has diluted out our true voice. The state doesn't accept our decisions. They're so used to making decisions for us.

If all the people voted for the strip searches, it should be possible. For example, they search passengers at the Anchorage airport. How is it any different in this village? Maybe the village should take their land back and run their own airport.

The issues in this case are self-determination, tribal sovereignty, self-government, and honoring our decision makers. As far as human rights, we're neglectful in Alaska. Our state government is too powerful. Just because a big city like Anchorage has more people and a large airport, people shouldn't penalize a small village.

Maybe they should let the state pull out. They could give money directly to the village, and they could hire their own staff directly, including their own public health nurse. The current system, with many staff at the regional level who "drop in" on the village to give itinerant services, is often not that responsive to the village needs. For example, requests for processing of grant monies that have already been received at the regional level, and are targeted for villages, may not get responded to very quickly. There's a "maybe I'll do it after Christmas" approach rather than an immediate response.

Methods should be looked at like contracting directly with the villages and giving them as much local control as possible, because they're the only ones who really care about their environment and community.

Example From Another Setting

Family Law in Papua New Guinea

In 1972, Papua New Guinea became an independent nation of 3.5 million people, speaking some 750 mutually unintelligible languages and living under a combination of a Western legal system that had been imposed by Australia and almost 1,000 different customary or traditional legal systems (Robbins 1993). The problems of reconciling customary law with the legal system imposed by Australia are illustrated by the legal changes that affected the Abelam. One Abelam man was jailed because he buried his deceased mother inside her house; custom required that a corpse be laid to rest in the house in which the person had worked and slept. The house would then be abandoned and eventually collapse around the burial site. Australian officials wanted this practice discontinued because they felt it constituted a health hazard.

Another legal problem was polygamy. Although most Abelam marriages were monogamous, some men had more than one wife. One elderly man with two wives expressed concern when he discovered that he was breaking the law, but he explained that he could never choose one wife over the other because he loved both. A family law bill was drafted to recognize customary marriages as legal and to allow polygamous marriages under certain conditions. Homicide compensation, traditionally paid to the aggrieved survivors, was another difficult issue. The payment, which was supposed to be proportionate to the act that caused the conflict, implied acceptance of responsibility by the donor and willingness to end the dispute by the recipient. These arrangements were not recognized under state law. In addition, the use of customary law changed as indigenous people came into contact with Western society. Some cases involved huge groups of people and claims of large compensatory payments. For example, when a man driving a truck struck and killed a man from another province, members of the victim's clan demanded hundreds of thousands of kina (currency equivalent to the Australian dollar) in compensation from the driver's whole province. After consultants made lawmakers aware of the cultural aspects of such situations, legislation was prepared to recognize the exchange of wealth and services as a means of resolving conflicts involving death, injuries, and property damage and to regulate payments by specifying the amount of compensation to be paid in specific circumstances but not setting limits on the competitive ceremonial exchanges.

Domestic violence was becoming a problem because of changing patterns of residence. Traditionally, after marriage, a woman went to live with her husband's family, but her own family would be nearby, and if she was abused by her husband she could return home. To obtain employment in developing areas, however, families often moved to other parts of the country, and wives could not return home easily. Special laws to help protect wives trapped in these situations needed to be developed.

9

Conclusions

The experiences of psychiatrists working in remote rural parts of Alaska are not unique. Similar cases, problems, and solutions can be found in many other places: in Third World developing countries, in rural areas of industrialized nations, and in some parts of the United States. The ideas and frameworks, the methods and techniques, are transferable to other cultures that may be at different stages of health transition, even if the specifics are not the same. A psychiatrist working in a Moslem country, for example, will not see the widespread problems connected with alcohol that are present in Alaska. However, the gaps between cultures, the importance of understanding community structure and dynamics, and the need to build trust and teamwork and to accomplish much with scant resources will be the same.

General Issues in Developing Areas

Major inequities exist in the distribution of resources between rich and poor countries and between urban and rural areas within countries (the so-called urban-rural divide). These inequities have general health impacts and mental health impacts. Among the indices that have been used to try to assess these impacts are caloric or protein intake, the number of doctors or health practitioners serving a particular segment of the population, the number of hours of work required to purchase basic commodities, life expectancy, infant mortality, and literacy. In most cases, developing areas, and remote rural areas within developed countries such as the Alaskan villages, come out poorly on these measurements.

In terms of health resources, some countries have 30 cents per person per year to spend on health, with less for the rural areas, and other countries have $3,000.00 or more. Effective access to government health services ranges widely: Some developing countries average one visit to the doctor per person every 10 years, whereas others average three to five visits a year. There may be one psychiatrist to cover 600,000 people, or better than one psychiatrist for every 8,000.

As for health research, 95% of the money used worldwide to study health problems is spent in the developed world. The distribution of research effort, like that of services, is highly skewed: 93% of the years of useful life lost are due to diseases in developing countries that receive only 5% of the world's health research funding. Decisions on how best to distribute limited resources are hampered when epidemiological data are lacking, and there is no statistical basis for attaching priority to health problems.

Expenditures in rural areas of developed countries are similarly skewed. Essential research directed toward understanding local problems, enhancing the impact of limited resources, improving health policy and management, fostering innovation and experimentation, providing the foundation for a stronger rural voice in setting priorities and policies, and improving the operation of services and programs is lacking. Clearly the paradigm for medical research in developing countries (as well as in rural areas of developed countries) needs to be changed or at least broadened (Anonymous 1990).

Until this happens, agenda will continue to be imposed by outside funding sources. However well intentioned, they tend insufficiently to involve indigenous people and to be categorical, piecemeal, and short term rather than interdisciplinary, broad based, and long term in outlook. This leads to a vicious circle of increasing problems and increasing neglect; rural and developing areas are considered peripheral or of limited interest and importance.

Yet the problems of urban areas and rural areas are intertwined in countless ways. For example, rural problems may lead to loss of a land base for the villagers, who then move into the cities to create problems such as shantytowns. To advance mental health programming for rural, developing areas, professionals must acknowledge the problems and must move away from the common tendencies to deny that the problems exist, or to define them as someone else's job, or to grasp at overly simplistic solutions.

General Development Strategies

Strategies that are currently being used in rural, developing areas are similar to those used in Alaska and described in this book. They include

1. Development of primary care networks. The primary care system focuses on health education, nutrition, water and sanitation, maternal and child health, immunization, control of communicable diseases, basic curative care provided by general practitioners or family physicians, and essential drugs (often with a simplified formulary). The mental health efforts attempt to build on the primary care system and the general hospitals and work closely with them.
2. Training of health personnel, including community health workers, focusing on the detection and management of psychiatric problems in primary care.
3. Population-based public health approaches, which involve targeting of high-risk groups.
4. Development of special programming to meet local needs, building on cultural strengths and using indigenous healers to augment the professional system.
5. Decentralization of services toward districts and villages.
6. Decentralized training, suited to primary care, with increasing specialization tailored to regional or national need.

Community Participation

The emphasis in many of these strategies is on broad-based community participation. The principles of community participation include

1. The community should decide in what form it will provide resources for health workers, including materials and labor.
2. The community should decide how to mobilize resources (e.g., user charges, assessments) rather than being handed a rigid system "from on high."
3. Preventative and educational services may be deferred, at least until a firm, broad demand base resting on personal experience of the value of these services has been built.
4. Cash raised at the community level should be spent there.

5. Communities should be encouraged to view health services, pure water, fuel, nutrition, and food security as interrelated; local government health personnel should receive training to help develop that approach.
6. Community-based catalysts for health promotion and education should be used.

Primary Health Care Approach

The primary health care approach has emerged in response to the growing realization that the supposed benefits of all the money spent on sophisticated curative medicine and hospital-centered, specialized care were not reaching the poor, mostly rural, populations that had the most disease. Assumptions that the wealthier countries had the capital, the talent, and the know-how to solve the health problems of the poorer countries have proven inadequate. Development of medical schools, hospitals, and clinics based on Western systems and the introduction of curative, hospital-centered care have, in fact, been particularly ill suited to some developing areas. Such health care is urban based, whereas the bulk of the population is rural. It is expensive, whereas the majority are poor. It is highly specialized and focused on esoteric diseases, whereas most rural people suffer from communicable diseases; deficiencies in sanitation; malnutrition; and, increasingly, lifestyle-related health problems associated with substance abuse, inadequate exercise, and unplanned pregnancies. The imported model of health care was imposed on the local systems without taking into account cultural or political realities.

The basic components that are now being stressed instead are community involvement; appropriate health technology; and reorientation of health services away from urban, hospital-based care toward country-wide health programs. Preventative medicine and use of community health workers to serve the needs of their communities are emphasized. Child survival is a priority; programs include growth monitoring, oral rehydration therapy, breast-feeding, improved weaning foods, immunization, food supplements, and family planning. Safe motherhood programs and attempts to decrease maternal mortality and improve women's reproductive health are also important, including stronger community-based care (such as use of traditional birth attendants), stronger referral facilities, and better transport systems for high-risk pregnancies.

The programs described in this book for rural Alaskan villages have been considerably influenced by these ideas. Many of the villages need basic sanitation, better nutrition, and improvements in housing. Maternal and child health programs have been a focus. Community health workers are used extensively, and local communities are encouraged to participate actively in their own health care. Prevention and health promotion strategies are emphasized, along with close cooperation with the existing primary care system.

Wider Implications

The Alaska material presented in this book reflects many of the concerns and problems experienced in other remote rural areas of the world. In Alaska, however, there are more resources to work with than in some other places, and a fascinating set of problems has been uncovered that up to now has received relatively little attention from the mental health community.

Each case presents a critical issue in a particular area, such as care for chronically mentally ill patients, use of primary care facilities and work with primary care physicians, strategies for developing new service systems, interprofessional staff differences, and family and cultural issues. Individuals with chronic mental illness who lack access to standard services, like Dog Bone in Case 1 (Chapter 2), and how to handle such patients in rural areas where resources are very scarce are major problems. So are the difficulties faced by small general hospitals, struggling to handle psychiatric emergencies without adequate staffing or facilities, as exemplified by the Outraged Nurse in Case 2 (Chapter 3).

Newly emerging health problems like fetal alcohol syndrome, which from a public health point of view require the development of a whole service system, are of increasing concern. Programs targeted at high-risk mothers and children with psychiatric disorders are expected to be part of a growing trend everywhere. A number of problems require the type of integrated response by multiple agencies and providers that Alaska is developing for children at risk for fetal alcohol syndrome. These problems include child abuse, child sexual abuse, childhood gasoline sniffing, teenage substance abuse, and suicidal behavior. The emphasis in many countries on child survival and on improving women's reproductive health means that psychiatric services will need to develop new ways to contribute.

Because of increasing globalization, topics considered in other chapters—the role of family support networks, cultural and language issues, and legal and socioeconomic concerns impacting on psychiatry—also seem likely to receive increasing interest and attention. The practice of psychiatry and psychiatrists' roles are likely to change dramatically. Interdisciplinary efforts with a variety of social scientists, as well as linkages with primary care systems, will be needed. Community health workers, being trained in many countries to provide frontline services at the village level, have until now worked mainly with physical health problems or as community health educators. Their potential for mental health work and how psychiatrists can best be involved in training or backup roles are issues that require considerable discussion. As some of the Alaska cases show, many problems that at first seem to be physical health issues have, on closer examination, behavioral lifestyle aspects. Team efforts that include psychiatrists can improve health outcomes in these kinds of problems.

Cultural issues can become evident when traditional beliefs are overlaid with varying combinations of ideas from missionary groups and current health beliefs from the non-Native medical system. Many subtle types of cultural identity problems can arise as formerly remote and isolated communities come into increasing contact with other parts of the world. The efforts in many countries to professionalize indigenous traditional healers as a way to leverage scarce professional resources, and how to do this with respect to psychiatric problems, could also benefit from increased discussion.

Other issues grow out of legal battles over fishing rights, land use, adoption policies, rights to local schooling, and numerous other topics. The Strip Search case in this book (Chapter 8) is just one variant on a common dynamic in which people attempt to achieve self-determination in ways that seem appropriate to them but that may not fit the laws of the dominant society. The public psychiatrist working with remote rural communities gets involved in such issues through, for example, testifying at hearings about the mental health impacts of various pieces of legislation or giving opinions on disposition in child custody and other types of civil cases in which lack of resources makes choices extremely difficult. Questions concerning the impact of environmental changes and pollution will likewise come increasingly to the fore as mental health activities are extended into previously unserved locations.

The cases in this book, therefore, represent just the tip of the iceberg. Psychiatric practice in remote rural areas has a widening circle of impacts and implications in the global community.

Realities and Rewards of Work in Remote Rural Locations

One of the purposes of this book is to encourage interest in a neglected area of psychiatry that has a lot of potential while acknowledging the realistic difficulties of working in underserved areas. Work in remote rural areas is among the most personally challenging, intellectually engaging, and potentially frustrating areas of psychiatry. On a personal level, it demands compassion and understanding in the midst of seemingly overwhelming disease, poverty, and suffering. An adequate understanding of the dynamics that lead to these conditions requires the integration of information from many spheres—biological, psychological, social, cultural, ecological, and others—using an array of methods ranging from anthropological-style fieldwork and participant observation to psycholinguistics to dealing with social, community, and cultural issues. Questions of professional boundaries, as well as broader political and economic forces, can play important parts in these situations, and what is presented often cannot be taken at face value. Unfortunately, theories and training to prepare psychiatrists adequately for this work are sadly lacking.

Adapting Ethnographic Methods

What could be called the "inner game" of remote rural consultation work includes thinking about the problems from new perspectives, considering various approaches to problem solving, and finding ways to learn more. Cognitive, problem-analysis, and observational skills can be developed and practiced. Yet self-observation, in which the psychiatrist attempts to become aware of his or her own deeply ingrained habits, expectations, and assumptions, may be even more important. Such self-observation can be difficult to teach because often the smarter and better educated a person is, the less willing he or she is to step back and ask seemingly obvious or stupid questions or to question activities that have been highly rewarded in the past. Close observation of others is of course also essential. Self-observation comes first, however, because without acute awareness of one's own assumptions and values, it is difficult to know what to look for in others. Some of the processes and techniques used by ethnographers in developing self-observation skills are well described by Bernard (1988).

Spradley (1979, 1980) and other ethnographers emphasize that to discover the cultural reality of a group of people, questions must be asked and meanings recorded in the local language. Learning the local terms and concepts is not simply acquiring the ability to communicate; it leads to discovering how natives categorize experience and how informants use these categories in customary thought. For Spradley, language is more than a means of communication about reality; it is a tool for constructing reality. Different languages categorize experience in different ways and provide alternative patterns for customary ways of thinking and perceiving.

The ethnographer, therefore, starts with a conscious attitude of almost complete ignorance—what can be called "maintaining naïveté." This runs counter to most professional training, where the goal is to render "expert" opinions. Instead of collecting "data" from people, or doing "studies" on them, or making "professional judgments," the ethnographer seeks to learn from people and be taught by them. Rather than testing formal theories developed elsewhere, the ethnographer attempts to formulate "grounded theory," rooted in empirical data of cultural description.

Within the field of psychiatry, further investigation of these topics could begin with the work of Murray Bowen (Papero 1988), as well as the Milan School of Systemic Family Therapy (Palazzoli 1983, 1984; Palazzoli et al. 1978, 1980a, 1980b; Penn 1982; Tomm 1984a, 1984b, 1987a, 1987b, 1988). These family therapists have extended their work to deal with larger systems, such as organizations, which are similar in some respects to villages and regions. Training curricula developed by followers of the Milan School can be very helpful to people learning the skills needed for working with remote rural groups.

The work of Kurt Lewin (1935, 1948), considered by many the father of social psychology, is still remarkably helpful. His ideas about action research, fields, topographic mapping, sensitivity training, and work on the social psychology of oppression of minority groups provide valuable orientation for people working in remote rural settings.

Organizing Information in Remote Rural Settings

The reason for doing all of this observing and questioning is to develop concentration and focused attention in dealing with what might be experienced as overwhelming, frustrating, and overly complex. This goes a long way to improving personal and professional effectiveness in unique settings where the ordinary rules do not always apply.

Establishing a method of organizing the mass of information that can be collected within a short time is essential. For complex problems, a "soft systems" approach can be helpful (Checkland and Scholes 1990). This approach was developed by planning and design experts and industrial engineers for complicated problems that have both quantitative and qualitative aspects; the vocabulary and approach must be general enough to cross boundaries so that they can be used in multiple settings and contexts to solve all types of problems. The soft systems approach described in the industrial engineering literature tries to define complicated systems problems in ways that permit various possible "solution options" to be considered. This is called "widening the potential solution space." Checkland and Scholes use a variety of diagramming techniques to analyze interactions and feedback loops, as well as potential ways to improve the system's functioning.

The average clinician tends to focus on a fairly standard set of treatment methods and to identify a limited number of types of "clients" and possible "agents." Little attention is usually paid to cultural and "world view" issues, to possible ways to achieve a more leveraged solution through changes at the management level, or to the full potential of collaboration with environmental forces (e.g., schools, courts).

The cases in this book present situations in which conventional methods would not work very well and describe attempts to alter or redefine one or several variables to reach workable solutions. This approach can be useful for all sorts of ill-structured and poorly defined problems.

Several schemes for organizing and systematically scanning large amounts of information are described earlier in this book. For example, Chapter 1 includes a health enhancement model; Chapter 3 describes a hospital system. All of these can be considered as special cases of Checkland and Scholes' (1990) general methodology. The health enhancement cube, for example, with its 36 compartments, defines who the client is (individual, interpersonal, something in the setting that might need to be modified), who and where the treatment agent is (individual/family, health care provider, school, work site, community), and what the treatment or change process might consist of (health behavior development, health behavior change, health behavior maintenance). The hospital system model focuses on the patients coming in (clients), the staff (agents of treatment), the treatment processes being used, the management or ownership issues, and so on.

The advantage of the more general model for psychiatrists is that it covers dimensions such as ownership and world view as well as standard types of operational questions about what is coming in, how it is getting processed, and who is doing what. In many of the cases in this book, there was room for disagreement about who should be responsible and "own" the problems and about basic values and how best to conceptualize and tackle the problems.

In Conclusion

Professional training programs leave psychiatric residents, as well as other mental health trainees, lacking in the necessary skills for work in remote rural settings; such skills include community consultation, social change interventions, and other alternatives to an individual approach. Courses on dealing with rural and culturally distinct clients are relegated to the periphery of the curriculum and tend to be seen as frills rather than core. Even the available world health literature concentrates on infectious diseases and infant mortality and pays relatively little attention to social and behavioral pathology. Clinical practicums and internships rarely deal with issues of empowerment, transformation, use of indigenous methods, natural support systems, development of lay helping networks, use of volunteers and extended family resources, collective treatments, or even public health approaches.

In view of this general lack in most training programs, the Group for the Advancement of Psychiatry members who went to Alaska spent a good deal of time discussing how best to process and organize what they had learned during their visits and how the information might usefully be communicated to trainees (e.g., psychiatric residents). Was there a way to help trainees better prepare for this type of work? Were there some general lessons from which even "mainstream" psychiatrists could benefit?

In the end, it was decided that the "casebook" format would provide readers with a sampling of real-life, experiential problems whose origins and solutions can be dissected and discussed. As health care reform progresses in many parts of the world, basic changes in assumptions and practices may be needed for everyone in the mental health professions. Psychiatric residents and other trainees have few opportunities for exposure to what is going on in psychiatry internationally. With increasing globalization, however, what used to be seen as remote will become a concern close to home.

The case examples and discussions are a poor substitute for actually going to work in a remote rural or developing country setting and experiencing it firsthand. However, because so few established researchers are currently studying these settings, and because almost no training materials are available, the cases in this book are at least a step in the right direction. This is a beginning, a scouting and mapping of relatively uncharted terrain. We hope it will generate enthusiasm and interest in exploring remote rural mental health issues.

In the coming years, as pressure grows on the health system to do more with less, the approaches and problem-solving strategies developed in underserved areas to deal with very limited resources will receive increasing attention. Mental health professionals will need to improve their abilities to become aware of their own assumptions, to define problems in innovative ways, to look for longer-term preventative solutions rather than short-term quick fixes, to recognize potentials for interdisciplinary team building and new types of staffing arrangements, and to deal with minorities and cultural diversity. These are the skills that are already being used and refined by psychiatrists in remote rural areas such as Alaska.

References

American Psychiatric Association: Diagnostic and Statistical Manual of Mental Disorders, 3rd Edition, Revised. Washington, DC, American Psychiatric Association, 1987

American Psychiatric Association: Diagnostic and Statistical Manual of Mental Disorders, 4th Edition. Washington, DC, American Psychiatric Association, 1994

Anonymous: Promoting health research for development. Lancet 336:1415–1416, 1990

Appleby L, Araya R: Mental Health Services in the Global Village (Royal College of Psychiatrists). London, England, Gaskell, 1991

Argyris C: Reasoning, Learning, and Action: Individual and Organizational. San Francisco, CA, Jossey-Bass, 1982

Argyris C: Strategy, Change, and Defensive Routines. Boston, MA, Pitman, 1985

Argyris C: Overcoming Organizational Defenses. Englewood Cliffs, NJ, Prentice-Hall, 1990

Bachrach L: Deinstitutionalization of mental health services in rural areas. Hosp Community Psychiatry 28:669–672, 1977

Bachrach L: The process of de-institutionalization in rural areas, in Handbook of Rural Mental Health, 1st Edition. Edited by Keller P, Murray J. New York, Human Sciences Press, 1982, pp 110–121

Bachrach L: Psychiatric services in rural areas: a sociological overview. Hosp Community Psychiatry 34:215–226, 1983

Barton G: The practice of emergency psychiatry in rural areas. Hosp Community Psychiatry 43:965–966, 1992

Bernard HR: Research Methods in Cultural Anthropology. Newbury Park, CA, Sage, 1988

Bisbee G: Management of Rural, Primary Care—Concepts and Cases. Chapel Hill, NC, Hospital Research and Educational Trust, 1982

Caldera D: Supervision of primary health care workers in Alaska: one approach, in Circumpolar Health 87: Proceedings of the 7th International Congress on Circumpolar Health, Umea, Sweden, June 8–12, 1987. Edited by Linderholm H, Backman C, Broadbent N, et al. Manitoba, Canada, University of Manitoba Press, 1988, pp 357–359

Caldera D, Daniels S, Ashenfelter W: The role of the community health aide in rural Alaska, in Circumpolar Health 90: Proceedings of the 8th International Congress on Circumpolar Health, Whitehorse, Yukon, May 20–25, 1990. Edited by Postl BD, Gilbert P, Goodwill J, et al. Manitoba, Canada, University of Manitoba Press, 1991, pp 157–160

Caldwell JC, Caldwell P, Gajanayake I, et al: Cultural, social, and behavioural determinants of health and their mechanisms: a report on related research programs, in What We Know About the Health Transition: The Proceedings of an International Workshop, Canberra, May 1989. Edited by Caldwell JC, Findley S, Caldwell P, et al. Canberra, Australia, Australian National University Press, 1990, pp 25–43

Checkland P, Scholes J: Soft Systems Methodology in Action. Chichester, England, Wiley, 1990

Chen L, Kleinman A, Ware N (eds): Advancing Health in Developing Countries: The Role of Social Research. New York, Auburn House, 1992

Craig R: Sivunniigvik (the Planning Place): Inupiat Ilitqusiat Program. Kotzebue, AK, NANA Museum of the Arctic, Quality Litho, 1988

Cutler D: Community-family network therapy in a rural setting. Community Ment Health J 16:144–155, 1980

D'Augelli A: Future directions for para-professionals in rural mental health, or how to avoid giving indigenous helpers civil service ratings, in Handbook of Rural Mental Health, 1st Edition. Edited by Keller P, Murray J. New York, Human Sciences Press, 1982, pp 210–222

Dubos R: Man Adapting. New Haven, CT, Yale University Press, 1965

Eguchi S: Between folk concepts of illness and psychiatric diagnosis: kitsune—tsuki (fox possession) in a mountain village of Western Japan. Cult Med Psychiatry 15:421–451, 1991

Fienup-Riordan A: Cultural Change and Identity Among Alaska Natives: Retaining Control. Anchorage, AK, Institute for Social and Economic Research, University of Alaska, Anchorage, 1992

Findley S: Introduction: addressing the health transition research agenda: can we connect findings with action? in Advancing Health in Developing Countries: The Role of Social Research. Edited by Chen L, Kleinman A, Ware N. New York, Auburn House, 1992, pp 1–22

Flanders N: Missionaries and professional infidels: religion and government in Western Alaska. Arctic Anthropology 28:44–62, 1991

Fleuridas C, Nelson TS, Rosenthal DM: The evolution of circular questions: training family therapists. Journal of Marital and Family Therapy 12:113–127, 1986

Fortuine R: The use of medicinal plants by the Alaska Natives. Alaska Med 30:185–226, 1988

Fortuine R: Chills and Fever: Health and Disease in the Early History of Alaska. Fairbanks, AK, University of Alaska Press, 1989

Fortuine R: The Health of the Inuit of North America: a Bibliography From the Earliest Times Through 1990. Anchorage, AK, University of Alaska, 1993

Francis M: The skeleton in the cupboard: experiential geneogram work for family therapy trainees. Journal of Family Therapy 10:135–152, 1988

Gabbard G: The treatment of the "special" patient in a psychoanalytic hospital. International Review of Psychoanalysis 13:333–347, 1986

Gaines A: Definitions and diagnoses: cultural implications of psychiatric help-seeking and psychiatrists' definitions of the situation in psychiatric emergencies. Cult Med Psychiatry 3:381–418, 1979

German GA: Mental Health in Africa, I: the extent of mental health problems in Africa today: an update of epidemiological knowledge, II: the nature of mental disorder in Africa today: some clinical observations. Br J Psychiatry 151:435–439, 1987

Giel R, Harding TW: Psychiatric priorities in developing countries. Br J Psychiatry 128:513–522, 1976

Goodluck C: Utilization of Genograms and Eco-Maps to Assess American Indian Families Who Have a Member with a Disability (Making Visible the Invisible): Training Curriculum. Flagstaff, AZ, American Indian Rehabilitation, Research & Training Center, Northern Arizona University, 1988

Green RH: Politics, power, and poverty: health for all in 2000 in the Third World? Soc Sci Med 32:745–755, 1991

Greene RJ, Mullen FG: A crisis telephone service in a nonmetropolitan area. Hosp Community Psychiatry 24:94–97, 1973

Halperin RH: Appalachians in cities: issues and challenges for research, in From Mountains to Metropolis: Appalachian Migrants in American Cities. Edited by Borman K, Obermiller P. Westport, CT, Greenwood, 1994, pp 65–80

Hartman A: A diagrammatic assessment of family relationships. Social Casework 59:465–476, 1978

Heinl P: The image and visual analysis of the geneogram. Journal of Family Therapy 7:213–229, 1985

Heinl P: Visual geneogram work and change: a single case study. Journal of Family Therapy 9:281–291, 1987

Helman C: Culture, Health and Illness, 2nd Edition. Stoneham, MA, Butterworth Heinemann, 1990

Helman C: Healer as ethnographer, ethnographer as healer. Paper presented at the 92nd annual meeting of the American Anthropological Association, Washington, DC, 1993

Herzberg F: Work and the Nature of Man. Cleveland, OH, World Publishing, 1966

Hoff W: Traditional healers as community health workers: a review of projects using traditional healers as community health workers (SHS/DHS/91.6). Geneva, Switzerland, World Health Organization, 1990

Hoff W: Traditional healers and community health. World Health Forum 13:182–187, 1992

Hoff W, Galowa K: Promoting Integral Human Development in the Community: A Manual for Trainers to Conduct Workshops for Community Leaders. Boroko, Papua, New Guinea, Department of Health, Environmental Health Section (PO Box 3991), 1989

Johnson T: Consultation psychiatry as applied medical anthropology, in Encounters With Biomedicine: Case Studies in Medical Anthropology. Edited by Baer H. New York, Gordon & Breach Science Publishers, 1987, pp 269–293

Jones L: The chronic mentally ill, in Psychiatric Services for Underserved Rural Populations. Edited by Jones L, Parlour R. New York, Brunner/Mazel, 1985, pp 280–293

Jones LR, Parlour R: Psychiatric Services for Underserved Rural Populations. New York, Brunner/Mazel, 1985

Kan S: The Russian Orthodox Church in Alaska, in Handbook of North American Indians, Vol 4: History of Indian-White Relations. Edited by Washburn W. Washington, DC, Smithsonian Institution, 1988, pp 506–521

Kapur RL: Mental health care in rural India: a study of existing patterns and their implications for future policy. Br J Psychiatry 127:286–293, 1975

Karp I: Deconstructing culture-bound syndromes. Soc Sci Med 21:221–228, 1985

Kates N: Training psychiatric residents to work with primary care physicians: results of a national survey. Can J Psychiatry 38:79–82, 1993

Keller P, Murray J (eds): Handbook of Rural Community Mental Health. New York, Human Sciences Press, 1982

Kim D: Systems Archetypes: Diagnosing Systemic Issues and Designing High-Leverage Interventions. Cambridge, MA, Pegasus Communications, 1992

Kleinman A: Patients and Healers in the Context of Culture. Berkeley, CA, University of California Press, 1980

Kleinman A: Anthropology and psychiatry: the role of culture in cross-cultural research on illness. Br J Psychiatry 151:447–454, 1987a

Kleinman A: Rethinking Psychiatry: From Cultural Category to Personal Experience. New York, Free Press, 1987b

Langsley D, Robinowitz C: Psychiatric manpower: an overview. Hosp Community Psychiatry 30:749–755, 1979

Leighton D, Harding J, Macklin D, et al: The Character of Danger: Psychiatric Symptoms in Selected Communities (The Stirling County Study of Psychiatric Disorders.) New York, Basic Books, 1963a

Leighton A, Lambo T, Hughes C, et al: Psychiatric Disorder Among the Yoruba. Ithaca, NY, Cornell University Press, 1963b

Lewin K: Dynamic Theory of Personality. New York, McGraw-Hill, 1935

Lewin K: Resolving social conflicts, in Selected Papers on Group Dynamics. Edited by Lewin GW. New York, Harper & Row, 1948

Libo L, Griffith C: Mental Health Consultants: Agents of Community Change, 1st Edition. San Francisco, CA, Jossey-Bass, 1968

McGoldrick M, Gerson R: Genograms in Family Assessment. New York, WW Norton, 1985

McNabb S: Elders, Inupiat Ilitqusiat, and culture goals in Northwest Alaska. Arctic Anthropology 28:63–76, 1991

Mead S, Stewart T, Cordes P, et al: A Family Wellness Needs Assessment for Alaska Head Start: Project Summary and Findings (Alaska Head Start Health Improvement Initiative). Anchorage, AK, Prevention Associates (101 E 9th Ave #10B, 99501), 1993

Mechanic D: Research possibilities on facilitating the health care transition, in Advancing Health in Developing Countries: The Role of Social Research. Edited by Chen L, Kleinman A, Ware N. New York, Auburn House, 1992, 49–56

Minuchin S: Family Therapy Techniques. Cambridge, MA, Harvard University Press, 1981

Minuchin S: Families and Family Therapy. London, England, Tavistock, 1982

Mohatt G, McDiarmid G, Montoya V: Societies, families, and change: the Alaskan example: behavioral health issues among American Indians and Alaska Natives. American Indian and Alaska Native Mental Health Research 1 (monograph no 1):325–365, 1987

Moxley D: The Practice of Case Management. Newbury Park, CA, Sage, 1989

Muller J: Managing professional socialization: lessons learned from medical students' encounters with attending physicians. Paper presented at the annual meeting of the American Anthropology Association, Washington, DC, November 1993

Murray J, Kupinsky S: The influence of powerlessness and natural support systems on mental health in the rural community, in Handbook of Rural Mental Health, 1st Edition. Edited by Keller P, Murray J. New York, Human Sciences Press, 1982, pp 62–73

O'Neil J: Colonial stress in the Canadian Arctic: an ethnography of young adults changing, in Anthropology and Epidemiology. Edited by Janes C, Stall R, Gifford S. Boston, MA, D Reidel, 1986

Palazzoli MS: The emergence of a comprehensive systems approach. Journal of Family Therapy 5:165–177, 1983

Palazzoli MS: Behind the scenes of the organization: some guidelines for the expert in human relations. Journal of Family Therapy 6:299–307, 1984

Palazzoli MS, Boscolo L, Cecchin GF, et al: Paradox and Counter-Paradox: A New Model in the Therapy of the Family in Schizophrenic Transaction. New York, Jason Aronson, 1978

Palazzoli MS, Boscolo L, Cecchin G, et al: Hypothesizing-circularity-neutrality: three guidelines for the conductor of the session. Fam Process 19:3–12, 1980a

Palazzoli MS, Boscolo L, Cecchin G, et al: The problem of the referring person. Journal of Marital and Family Therapy 6:3–9, 1980b

Papero DV: Training in Bowen theory, in Handbook of Family Therapy Training and Supervision. Edited by Liddle HA, Breunlin DC, Schwartz RC. New York, Guilford, 1988, pp 85–98

Pathman DE, Konrad TR, Ricketts TC III: The comparative retention of National Health Service Corps and other rural physicians: results of a 9-year follow-up study. JAMA 268:1552–1558, 1992

Penn P: Circular questioning. Fam Process 20:267–280, 1982

President's Commission on Mental Health: Report to the President, Vol 1. Washington, DC, U.S. Government Printing Office, 1978

Preston J, Brown FW, Hartley B: Using telemedicine to improve health care in distant areas. Hosp Community Psychiatry 43:25–32, 1992

Prince R, Tcheng-Laroche F: Culture-bound syndromes and international disease classifications. Cult Med Psychiatry 11:3–19, 1987

Prucha F: Two roads to conversion: Protestant and Catholic missionaries in the Pacific Northwest. Pacific Northwest Quarterly 79:130–137, 1988

Quick R, Bashshur R: Three perspectives on community health aides: surveys of health aides, consumers, and providers in western Alaska, in Circumpolar Health 90: Proceedings of the 8th International Congress on Circumpolar Health, Whitehorse, Yukon, May 20–25, 1990. Edited by Postl BD, Gilbert P, Goodwill J, et al. Manitoba, Canada, University of Manitoba Press, 1991, pp 161–165

Rabinowitz HK: Recruitment, retention, and follow-up of graduates of a program to increase the number of family physicians in rural and underserved areas. N Engl J Med 328:934–939, 1993

Robbins R: Cultural Anthropology: A Problem-Based Approach. Itasca, IL, Peacock, 1993

Ruvinni U: Networking Families in Crisis. New York, Human Sciences Press, 1978

Samson D: Villages flout the Constitution to keep drugs and alcohol out. Anchorage Daily News, November 11, 1992, pp B1–3

Sandler I, Lakey B: Locus of control as a stress moderator: the role of control perceptions of social support. Am J Community Psychol 10:65–80, 1982

Santos AB, Deci PA, La Chance KR, et al: Providing assertive community treatment for severely mentally ill patients in a rural area. Hosp Community Psychiatry 44:34–39, 1993

Sawyer C, Sawyer D: The malaria transition and the role of social science research, in Advancing Health in Developing Countries: The Role of Social Research. Edited by Chen L, Kleinman A, Ware N. New York, Auburn House, 1992, pp 105–122

Schatzman L, Strauss A: Field Research: Strategies for a Natural Sociology. Englewood Cliffs, NJ, Prentice Hall, 1973

Scherkenback W: The Deming Route to Quality and Productivity. Washington, DC, Ceep Press, 1986

Senge P: The Fifth Discipline: The Art and Practice of the Learning Organization, 1st Edition. New York, Doubleday/Currency, 1990a

Senge P: The leader's new work: building learning organizations. Sloan Management Review 32:7–23, 1990b

Speck R, Attneave C: Family Networks. New York, Vintage Books, 1973

Spradley J: The Ethnographic Interview. New York, Holt, Rinehart & Winston, 1979

Spradley JP: Participant Observation. New York, Holt, Rinehart & Winston, 1980

Streather A: Summary: International Workshop on Indigenous Knowledge and Community-Based Resource Management, Winnipeg, Manitoba, Canada, September 24–26, 1991. Ottawa, Canada, ECO-ED, 1991

Tan M, Querubin M, Rilloria T: The integration of traditional medicine among community-based health programmes in the Phillipines. J Trop Pediatr 2:71–74, 1988

Tomm K: One perspective on the Milan systemic approach, 1: overview of development, theory and practice. Journal of Marital and Family Therapy 10:113–125, 1984a

Tomm K: One perspective on the Milan systemic approach, 2: description of session format, interviewing style and interventions. Journal of Marital and Family Therapy 10:253–271, 1984b

Tomm K: Interventive interviewing, I: strategizing as a fourth guideline for the therapist. Fam Process 26:3–13, 1987a

Tomm K: Interventive interviewing, II: reflexive questioning as a means to enable self-healing. Fam Process 26:167–183, 1987b

Tomm K: Interventive interviewing, III: intending to ask lineal, circular, strategic, or reflexive questions? Fam Process 27:1–15, 1988

Van Stone J: Some aspects of religious change among Native inhabitants in West Alaska and the Northwest Territories. Arctic Anthropology 2:21–24, 1964

Weiss S: Behavioral medicine, health behavior, and health maintenance strategies: applicability to disease prevention in the developing world, in Advancing Health in Developing Countries: The Role of Social Research. Edited by Chen L, Kleinman A, Ware N. New York, Auburn House, 1992, pp 39–48

Whyte K: Aboriginal rights: the Native Americans' struggle for survival. Human Organizations 41:178–184, 1982

Will D, Baird D: An integrated approach to dysfunction in interprofessional systems. Journal of Family Therapy 6:275–290, 1984

GAP Committees and Membership

Committee on Adolescence

Richard C. Marohn, Chicago, IL, *Chairperson*
Ian A. Canino, New York, NY
Warren J. Gadpaille, Denver, CO
Harvey Horowitz, Philadelphia, PA
Sarah Huertas-Goldman, San Juan, PR
Paulina F. Kernberg, New York, NY
Clarice J. Kestenbaum, New York, NY
Silvio J. Onesti, Jr., Belmont, MA

Committee on Aging

Gene D. Cohen, Washington, DC, *Chairperson*
Karen Blank, West Hartford, CT
Charles M. Gaitz, Houston, TX
Gary Gottlieb, Philadelphia, PA
Ira R. Katz, Philadelphia, PA
Andrew F. Leuchter, Los Angeles, CA
Gabe J. Maletta, Minneapolis, MN
Richard A. Margolin, Nashville, TN
Kenneth M. Sakauye, New Orleans, LA
Charles A. Shamoian, Larchmont, NY
F. Conyers Thompson, Jr., Atlanta, GA

Committee on Alcoholism and the Addictions

Joseph Westermeyer, Minneapolis, MN, *Chairperson*
Richard J. Frances, Newark, NJ
William Frosch, New York, NY
Marc Galanter, New York, NY
Earl A. Loomis, Jr., Augusta, GA
Robert Millman, New York, NY
Edgar P. Nace, Dallas, TX
Richard Suchinsky, Silver Spring, MD
Doug Ziedonis, New Haven, CT
John S. Tamerin, Greenwich, CT

Committee on Child Psychiatry

Peter Jensen, *Co-Chairperson*
David A. Mrazek, Denver, CO, *Co-Chairperson*
James M. Bell, Canaan, NY
Harlow Donald Dunton, New York, NY
Joseph Fischhoff, Detroit, MI
Joseph M. Green, Madison, WI
John F. McDermott, Jr., Honolulu, HI
Cynthia R. Pfeffer, White Plains, NY
John Schowalter, New Haven, CT
Theodore Shapiro, New York, NY
Peter E. Tanguay, Los Angeles, CA
Leonore Terr, San Francisco, CA

Committee on College Students

Earle Silber, Chevy Chase, MD, *Chairperson*
Robert L. Arnstein, Hamden, CT
Varda Backus, La Jolla, CA
Harrison P. Eddy, New York, NY
Myron B. Liptzin, Chapel Hill, NC
Malkah Tolpin Notman, Brookline, MA
Gloria C. Onque, Pittsburgh, PA
Elizabeth Aub Reid, Cambridge, MA
Lorraine D. Siggins, New Haven, CT
Tom G. Stauffer, White Plains, NY

Committee on Cultural Psychiatry

Ezra Griffith, New Haven, CT, *Chairperson*
Edward Foulks, New Orleans, LA
Francis Lu, San Francisco, CA
Pedro Ruiz, Houston, TX
Ronald Wintrob, Providence, RI
Joe Yamamoto, Los Angeles, CA

Committee on Disabilities

Meyer S. Gunther, Chicago, IL, *Chairperson*
Bryan King, Los Angeles, CA
Robert S. Nesheim, Duluth, MN
William H. Sack, Portland, OR
William A. Sonis, Philadelphia, PA
Margaret L. Stuber, Los Angeles, CA
Henry H. Work, Bethesda, MD

Committee on the Family

Frederick Gottlieb, Los Angeles, CA, *Chairperson*
W. Robert Beavers, Dallas, TX
Henry U. Grunebaum, Cambridge, MA
Herta A. Guttman, Montreal, PQ
Judith Landau-Stanton, Rochester, NY
Ann L. Price, Avon, CT

Committee on Government Policy

Roger Peele, Washington, DC, *Chairperson*
Thomas L. Clannon, San Francisco, CA
Naomi Heller, Washington, DC
John P. D. Shemo, Charlottesville, VA
William W. Van Stone, Washington, DC
Alan Zientes, Washington, DC

Committee on Human Sexuality

Bertram H. Schaffner, New York, NY, *Chairperson*
Paul L. Adams, Louisville, KY

Altha Stewart, New York, NY
Michael Vergare, Philadelphia, PA
George F. Wilson, Somerville, NJ
Jack A. Wolford, Pittsburgh, PA

Committee on Occupational Psychiatry

David B. Robbins, Chappaqua, NY, *Chairperson*
Peter L. Brill, Radnor, PA
Barrie S. Greiff, Newton, MA
Duane Q. Hagen, St. Louis, MO
R. Edward Huffman, Asheville, NC
Robert Larsen, San Francisco, CA
David E. Morrison, Palatine, IL
Jay B. Rohrlich, New York, NY
Clarence J. Rowe, St. Paul, MN
Jeffrey L. Speller, Cambridge, MA

Committee on Planning and Communications

Robert W. Gibson, Towson, MD, *Chairperson*
C. Knight Aldrich, Charlottesville, VA
Allan Beigel, Tucson, AZ
Doyle I. Carson, Dallas, TX
Paul J. Fink, Philadelphia, PA
Robert S. Garber, Longboat Key, FL
Harvey L. Ruben, New Haven, CT
Melvin Sabshin, Washington, DC
Michael R. Zales, Tucson, AZ

Committee on Preventive Psychiatry

Naomi Rae-Grant, London, ON, *Chairperson*
Viola W. Bernard, New York, NY
Stephen Fleck, New Haven, CT
Brian J. McConville, Cincinnati, OH
David R. Offord, Hamilton, ON
Morton M. Silverman, Chicago, IL
Warren T. Vaughan, Jr., Portola Valley, CA

Robert A. Dorwart, Cambridge, MA
James M. Ellison, Watertown, MA
Howard H. Goldman, Potomac, MD
Samuel G. Siris, Glen Oaks, NY

Committee on Public Education

Steven E. Katz, New York, NY, *Chairperson*
David Baron, Ambler, PA
Jack W. Bonner III, Asheville, NC
Jeffrey L. Geller, Worcester, MA
Jeanne Leventhal, Hayward, CA
David Preven, New York, NY
Elise K. Richman, Scarsdale, NY
Boris G. Rifkin, Branford, CT
Andrew E. Slaby, Summit, NJ
Robert A. Solow, Los Angeles, CA
Calvin R. Sumner, Buckhannon, WV
Laurence Tancredi, New York, NY

Committee on Research

Zebulon Taintor, New York, NY, *Chairperson*
Robert Cancro, New York, NY
Russell Gardner, Galveston, TX
John H. Greist, Madison, WI
Jerry M. Lewis, Dallas, TX
John G. Looney, Durham, NC

Committee on Social Issues

Martha J. Kirkpatrick, Los Angeles, CA, *Chairperson*
Ian E. Alger, New York, NY
William R. Beardslee, Waban, MA
Roderic Gorney, Los Angeles, CA
H. James Lurie, Seattle, WA
Ted Nadelson, Boston, MA
Perry Ottenberg, Philadelphia, PA
Kendon W. Smith, Pearl River, NY

Committee on Therapeutic Care

Alan Gruenberg, Philadelphia, PA, *Chairperson*
Bernard Bandler, Cambridge, MA
Thomas E. Curtis, Chapel Hill, NC
Donald C. Fidler, Morgantown, WV
Donald W. Hammersley, Washington, DC
William B. Hunter III, Albuquerque, NM
Milton Kramer, Cincinnati, OH
John Lipkin, Perry Point, MA
William W. Richards, Anchorage, AK

Committee on Therapy

Susan Lazar, Washington, DC, *Chairperson*
Gerald Adler, Boston, MA
Jules R. Bemporad, White Plains, NY
Eugene B. Feigelson, Brooklyn, NY
Andrew P. Morrison, Cambridge, MA
William C. Offenkrantz, Scottsdale, AZ
Allan D. Rosenblatt, La Jolla, CA
Robert Waldinger, West Newton, MA

GINSBURG FELLOWS

Arlener Artis-Trower, Silver Spring, MD *(Committee on Therapeutic Care)*
Elizabeth C. Druss, Cambridge, MA *(Committee on Psychopathology)*
Louis Michel Elie, LaSalle, Quebec, Canada *(Committee on Aging)*
Ryan Finkenbine, Charleston, SC *(Committee on Social Issues)*
Risa Fishman, New York, NY *(Committee on Alcoholism and the Addictions)*
Anna Lucy Fitzgerald, Brighton, MA *(Committee on Cultural Psychiatry)*
Michael Golding, Carrboro, NC *(Committee on Government Policy)*
Scott A. Haas, Louisville, KY *(Committee on Psychiatry and the Law)*
Jacqueline Haimes, Silver Spring, MD *(Committee on Planning and Communications)*
Samia Hasan, Baltimore, MD *(Committee on College Students)*
Lyudmila Karlin, Great Neck, NY *(Committee on Psychiatry and the Community)*
Vassilis Koliatsos, Baltimore, MD *(Committee on Research)*
Heather Krell, Philadelphia, PA *(Committee on Disabilities)*

Patricia Lester, San Francisco, CA *(Committee on Adolescence)*
Mercedes Martinez, Chicago, IL *(Committee on Child Psychiatry)*
Michael Fuller McBride, Milwaukee, WI *(Committee on Public Education)*
Alan Newman, Little Rock, AR *(Committee on International Relations)*
Robert Rogan, Greenville, NC *(Committee on Occupational Psychiatry)*
Jennifer Felice Schreiber, New York, NY *(Committee on Medical Education)*
Roseanne State, Pacific Palisades, CA *(Committee on Therapy)*
Teresa M. Stathas, Columbia, SC *(Committee on Psychiatry and Religion)*
Lynelle Thomas, New Haven, CT *(Committee on Preventive Psychiatry)*
Anna Viltz, Houston, TX *(Committee on Human Sexuality)*
Kenneth William Wilson, New York, NY *(Committee on Mental Health Services)*
Larry Wissow, Baltimore, MD *(Committee on the Family)*

CONTRIBUTING MEMBERS

Gene Abroms, Ardmore, PA
Carlos C. Alden, Jr., Buffalo, NY
Kenneth Z. Altshuler, Dallas, TX
Francis F. Barnes, Washington, DC
Spencer Bayles, Houston, TX
C. Christian Beels, New York, NY
Elissa P. Benedek, Ann Arbor, MI
Renee L. Binder, San Francisco, CA
Mark Blotcky, Dallas, TX
H. Keith H. Brodie, Durham, NC
Charles M. Bryant, San Francisco, CA
Ewald W. Busse, Durham, NC
Robert N. Butler, New York, NY
Eugene M. Caffey, Jr., Bowie, MD
Robert J. Campbell, New York, NY
James P. Cattell, San Diego, CA
Ian L. W. Clancey, Maitland, ON
Sanford I. Cohen, Coral Gables, FL
Lee Combrinck-Graham, Evanston, IL
Robert E. Drake, Hanover, NH
James S. Eaton, Jr., Washington, DC
Lloyd C. Elam, Nashville, TN
Joseph T. English, New York, NY

Sherman C. Feinstein, Highland Park, IL
Archie R. Foley, New York, NY
Henry J. Gault, Highland Park, IL
Richard K. Goodstein, Belle Mead, NJ
*Alexander Gralnick, Port Chester, NY
Milton Greenblatt, Sylmar, CA
Lawrence F. Greenleigh, Los Angeles, CA
Stanley I. Greenspan, Bethesda, MD
Jon E. Gudeman, Milwaukee, WI
William Hetznecker, Merion Station, PA
Johanna A. Hoffman, Scottsdale, AZ
Edward J. Khantzian, Haverhill, MA
James A. Knight, New Orleans, LA
Othilda M. Krug, Cincinnati, OH
Anthony F. Lehman, Baltimore, MD
Alan I. Levenson, Tucson, AZ
Norman L. Loux, Sellersville, PA
Albert J. Lubin, Woodside, CA
John Mack, Chestnut Hill, MA
John A. MacLeod, Cincinnati, OH
Charles A. Malone, Barrington, RI
Peter A. Martin, Lake Orion, MI
Alan A. McLean, Gig Harbor, WA
David Mendell, Houston, TX
Mary E. Mercer, Nyack, NY
Derek Miller, Chicago, IL
Steven M. Mirin, Belmont, MA
Richard D. Morrill, Boston, MA
Robert J. Nathan, Philadelphia, PA
Joseph D. Noshpitz, Washington, DC
Mortimer Ostow, Bronx, NY
Bernard L. Pacella, New York, NY
Herbert Pardes, New York, NY
Norman L. Paul, Lexington, MA
Marvin E. Perkins, Salem, VA
George H. Pollock, Chicago, IL
Becky Potter, Tucson, AZ

---

* Deceased.

David N. Ratnavale, Bethesda, MD
W. Donald Ross, Cincinnati, OH
Loren Roth, Pittsburgh, PA
Charles Shagass, Philadelphia, PA
Albert J. Silverman, Ann Arbor, MI
Benson R. Snyder, Cambridge, MA
David A. Soskis, Bala Cynwyd, PA
Jeffrey L. Speller, Cambridge, MA
Jeanne Spurlock, Washington, DC
Brandt F. Steele, Denver, CO
Alan A. Stone, Cambridge, MA
Perry C. Talkington, Dallas, TX
John A. Talbott, Baltimore, MD
Bryce Templeton, Philadelphia, PA
Prescott W. Thompson, Portland, OR
John A. Turner, San Francisco, CA
Andrew S. Watson, Ann Arbor, MI
Paul Tyler Wilson, Bethesda, MD
Ann Marie Wolf-Schatz, Conshohocken, PA
Kent A. Zimmerman, Menlo Park, CA
Howard Zonana, New Haven, CT

LIFE MEMBERS

C. Knight Aldrich, Charlottesville, VA
Robert L. Arnstein, Hamden, CT
Bernard Bandler, Cambridge, MA
Walter E. Barton, Hartland, VT
Viola W. Bernard, New York, NY
Henry W. Brosin, Tucson, AZ
John Donnelly, Hartford, CT
Merrill T. Eaton, Omaha, NE
O. Spurgeon English, Narberth, PA
Stephen Fleck, New Haven, CT
Jerome Frank, Baltimore, MD
Robert S. Garber, Longboat Key, FL
Robert I. Gibson, Towson, MD
Margaret M. Lawrence, Pomona, NY
Jerry M. Lewis, Dallas, TX
Harold I. Lief, Philadelphia, PA

Judd Marmor, Los Angeles, CA
Herbert C. Modlin, Topeka, KS
John C. Nemiah, Hanover, NH
William C. Offenkrantz, Scottsdale, AZ
Mabel Ross, Sun City, AZ
Julius Schreiber, Washington, DC
Robert E. Switzer, Dunn Loring, VA
Jack A. Wolford, Pittsburgh, PA
Henry H. Work, Bethesda, MD
Michael R. Zales, Tucson, AZ

BOARD OF DIRECTORS

Officers

President
Doyle I. Carson
P.O. Box 28218
Dallas, TX   75228

President-Elect
Malkah T. Notman
The Cambridge Hospital
54 Clark Road
Brookline, MA   02146

Secretary
Stephen C. Scheiber
ABPN
500 Lake Cook Road
Deerfield, IL   60015

Treasurer
Jack W. Bonner III
Behavioral Health Services
701 Grove Road
Greenville, SC   29605

Board Members
Ian Alger
Gene Cohen

Leah Dickstein
José Santiago

Past Presidents
*William C. Menninger   1946–51
Jack R. Ewalt   1951–53
Walter E. Barton   1953–55
*Sol W. Ginsburg   1955–57
*Dana L. Farnsworth   1957–59
*Marion E. Kenworthy   1959–61
Henry W. Brosin   1961–63
*Leo H. Bartemeier   1963–65
Robert S. Garber   1965–67
Herbert C. Modlin   1967–69
John Donnelly   1969–71
George Tarjan   1971–73
Judd Marmor   1973–75
John C. Nemiah   1975–77
Jack A. Wolford   1977–79
Robert W. Gibson   1979–81
*Jack Weinberg   1981–82
Henry H. Work   1982–85
Michael R. Zales   1985–87
Jerry M. Lewis   1987–89
Carolyn B. Robinowitz   1989–91
Allan Beigel   1991–93
John Schowalter   1993– 95

PUBLICATIONS BOARD

Chairperson
Allan Beigel
P.O. Box 43460
Tucson, AZ   85733

C. Knight Aldrich
Robert L. Arnstein

---

* Deceased.

Ezra Griffith
Steve Katz
W. Walter Menninger

Consultants
John C. Nemiah
Henry H. Work

Ex-Officio
John Schowalter
Carolyn B. Robinowitz

CONTRIBUTORS

Bristol Myers Squibb Company
Burroughs Wellcome Company
Glaxo, Inc.
GLS Associates, Inc.
Edith F. Goldensohn
Murel Foundation
Phillips Foundation
PRMS
The Upjohn Company
Westinghouse Electric Corporation
Wyeth-Ayerst Laboratories

GAP Publications

Mental Health in Remote Rural Developing Areas: Concepts and Cases (GAP Report 139, 1995), Formulated by the Committee on Therapeutic Care

Introduction to Occupational Psychiatry (GAP Report 138, 1994), Formulated by the Committee on Occupational Psychiatry

Forced Into Treatment: The Role of Coercion in Clinical Practice (GAP Report 137, 1994), Formulated by the Committee on Government Policy

Resident's Guide to Treatment of People With Chronic Mental Illness (GAP Report 136, 1993), Formulated by the Committee on Psychiatry and the Community

Caring for People With Physical Impairment: The Journey Back (GAP Report 135, 1992), Formulated by the Committee on Handicaps

Beyond Symptom Suppression: Improving Long-Term Outcomes of Schizophrenia (GAP Report 134, 1992), Formulated by the Committee on Psychopathology

Psychotherapy in the Future (GAP Report 133, 1992), Formulated by the Committee on Therapy

---

*Title is out of print.
†Available from Books on Demand, University Microfilms International, 300 North Zeeb Road, Ann Arbor, MI 48106-1346 (800-521-0600, ext. 3492).

Leaders and Followers: A Psychiatric Perspective on Religious Cults (GAP Report 132, 1992), Formulated by the Committee on Psychiatry and Religion

The Mental Health Professional and the Legal System (GAP Report 131, 1991), Formulated by the Committee on Psychiatry and the Law

*Psychotherapy With College Students (GAP Report 130, 1990), Formulated by the Committee on the College Student

A Casebook in Psychiatric Ethics (GAP Report 129, 1990), Formulated by the Committee on Medical Education

*Suicide and Ethnicity in the United States (GAP Report 128, 1989), Formulated by the Committee on Cultural Psychiatry

Psychiatric Prevention and the Family Life Cycle: Risk Reduction by Frontline Practitioners (GAP Report 127, 1989), Formulated by the Committee on Preventive Psychiatry

How Old Is Old Enough? The Ages of Rights and Responsibilities (GAP Report 126, 1989), Formulated by the Committee on Child Psychiatry

The Psychiatric Treatment of Alzheimer's Disease (GAP Report 125, 1988), Formulated by the Committee on Aging

Speaking Out for Psychiatry: A Handbook for Involvement With the Mass Media (GAP Report 124, 1987), Formulated by the Committee on Public Education

Us and Them: The Psychology of Ethnonationalism (GAP Report 123, 1987), Formulated by the Committee on International Relations

Psychiatry and Mental Health Professionals (GAP Report 122, 1987), Formulated by the Committee on Governmental Agencies

Interactive Fit: A Guide to Nonpsychotic Chronic Patients (GAP Report 121, 1987), Formulated by the Committee on Psychopathology

Teaching Psychotherapy in Contemporary Psychiatric Residency Training (GAP Report 120, 1986), Formulated by the Committee on Therapy

A Family Affair: Helping Families Cope With Mental Illness: A Guide for the Professions (GAP Report 119, 1986), Formulated by the Committee on Psychiatry and the Community

Crises of Adolescence—Teenage Pregnancy: Impact on Adolescent Development (GAP Report 118, 1986), Formulated by the Committee on Adolescence

The Family, the Patient, and the Psychiatric Hospital: Toward a New Model (GAP Report 117, 1985), Formulated by the Committee on Family

*†**Research and the Complex Causality of the Schizophrenias** (GAP Report 116, 1984), Formulated by the Committee on Research

***Friends and Lovers in the College Years** (GAP Report 115, 1983), Formulated by the Committee on the College Student

***Mental Health and Aging: Approaches to Curriculum Development** (GAP Report 114, 1983), Formulated by the Committee on Aging

Community Psychiatry: A Reappraisal (GAP Report 113, 1983), Formulated by the Committee on Psychiatry and the Community

The Child and Television Drama (GAP Report 112, 1982), Formulated by the Committee on Social Issues

***The Process of Child Therapy** (GAP Report 111, 1982), Formulated by the Committee on Child Psychiatry

The Positive Aspects of Long-Term Hospitalization in the Public Sector for Chronic Psychiatric Patients (GAP Report 110, 1982), Formulated by the Committee on Psychopathology

Job Loss—A Psychiatric Perspective (GAP Report 109, 1982), Formulated by the Committee on Psychiatry in Industry

A Survival Manual for Medical Students (GAP Report 108, 1982), Formulated by the Committee on Medical Education

INTERFACES: A Communication Casebook for Mental Health Decision Makers (GAP Report 107, 1981), Formulated by the Committee on Mental Health Services

***Divorce, Child Custody and the Family** (GAP Report 106, 1980), Formulated by the Committee on Family

***Mental Health and Primary Medical Care** (GAP Report 105, 1980), Formulated by the Committee on Preventive Psychiatry

Psychiatric Consultation in Mental Retardation (GAP Report 104, 1979), Formulated by the Committee on Mental Retardation

***Self-Involvement in the Middle East Conflict** (GAP Report 103, 1978), Formulated by the Committee on International Relations

The Chronic Mental Patient in the Community (GAP Report 102, 1978), Formulated by the Committee on Psychiatry and the Community

Power and Authority in Adolescence: The Origins and Resolutions of Intergenerational Conflict (GAP Report 101, 1978), Formulated by the Committee on Adolescence

***Psychotherapy and Its Financial Feasibility Within the National Health Care System** (GAP Report 100, 1978), Formulated by the Committee on Therapy

*†**What Price Compensation?** (GAP Report 99, 1977), Formulated by the Committee on Psychiatry in Industry

*Psychiatry and Sex Psychopath Legislation: The 30s to the 80s (GAP
   Report 98, 1977), Formulated by the Committee on Psychiatry and Law
Mysticism: Spiritual Quest or Psychic Disorder? (GAP Report 97, 1976),
   Formulated by the Committee on Psychiatry and Religion
*†Recertification: A Look at the Issues (GAP Report 96, 1976), Formu-
   lated by the Ad hoc Committee on Recertification
*†The Effect of the Method of Payment on Mental Health Care Practice
   (GAP Report 95, 1975), Formulated by the Committee on Govern-
   mental Agencies
*The Psychiatrist and Public Welfare Agencies (GAP Report 94, 1975),
   Formulated by the Committee on Psychiatry and the Community
*Pharmacotherapy and Psychotherapy: Paradoxes, Problems and Prog-
   ress (GAP Report 93, 1975), Formulated by the Committee on Research
*The Educated Woman: Prospects and Problems (GAP Report 92, 1975),
   Formulated by the Committee on the College Student
*†The Community Worker: A Response to Human Need (GAP Report
   91, 1974), Formulated by the Committee on Therapeutic Care
*†Problems of Psychiatric Leadership (GAP Report 90, 1974), Formu-
   lated by the Committee on Therapy
*Misuse of Psychiatry in the Criminal Courts: Competency to Stand
   Trial (GAP Report 89, 1974), Formulated by the Committee on Psy-
   chiatry and Law
Assessment of Sexual Function: A Guide to Interviewing (GAP Report
   88, 1973), Formulated by the Committee on Medical Education
From Diagnosis to Treatment: An Approach to Treatment Planning for
   the Emotionally Disturbed Child (GAP Report 87, 1973), Formu-
   lated by the Committee on Child Psychiatry
*†Humane Reproduction (GAP Report 86, 1973), Formulated by the
   Committee on Preventive Psychiatry
*The Welfare System and Mental Health (GAP Report 85, 1973), Formu-
   lated by the Committee on Psychiatry and Social Work
*†The Joys and Sorrows of Parenthood (GAP Report 84, 1973), Formu-
   lated by the Committee on Public Education
*The VIP With Psychiatric Impairment (GAP Report 83, 1973), Formu-
   lated by the Committee on Governmental Agencies
*Crisis in Child Mental Health: A Critical Assessment (GAP Report 82,
   1972), Formulated by the Ad hoc Committee
The Aged and Community Mental Health: A Guide to Program Development (GAP Report 81, 1971), Formulated by the Committee on
   Aging

*Drug Misuse: A Psychiatric View of a Modern Dilemma (GAP Report 80, 1970), Formulated by the Committee on Mental Health Services

*†Toward a Public Policy on Mental Health Care of the Elderly (GAP Report 79, 1970), Formulated by the Committee on Aging

The Field of Family Therapy (GAP Report 78, 1970), Formulated by the Committee on Family

*Toward Therapeutic Care (2nd Edition—No. 51 revised) (GAP Report 77, 1970), Formulated by the Committee on Therapeutic Care

*The Case History Method in the Study of Family Process (GAP Report 76, 1970), Formulated by the Committee on Family

*The Right to Abortion: A Psychiatric View (GAP Report 75, 1969), Formulated by the Committee on Psychiatry and Law

*†The Psychiatrist and Public Issues (GAP Report 74, 1969), Formulated by the Committee on International Relations

*†Psychotherapy and the Dual Research Tradition (GAP Report 73, 1969), Formulated by the Committee on Therapy

*Crisis in Psychiatric Hospitalization (GAP Report 72, 1969), Formulated by the Committee on Therapeutic Care

*On Psychotherapy and Casework (GAP Report 71, 1969), Formulated by the Committee on Psychiatry and Social Work

*The Nonpsychotic Alcoholic Patient and the Mental Hospital (GAP Report 70, 1968), Formulated by the Committee on Mental Health Services

*The Dimensions of Community Psychiatry (GAP Report 69, 1968), Formulated by the Committee on Preventive Psychiatry

*Normal Adolescence (GAP Report 68, 1968), Formulated by the Committee on Adolescence

The Psychic Function of Religion in Mental Illness and Health (GAP Report 67, 1968), Formulated by the Committee on Psychiatry and Religion

*Mild Mental Retardation: A Growing Challenge to the Physician (GAP Report 66, 1967), Formulated by the Committee on Mental Retardation

*†The Recruitment and Training of the Research Psychiatrist (GAP Report 65, 1967), Formulated by the Committee on Psychopathology

*Education for Community Psychiatry (GAP Report 64, 1967), Formulated by the Committee on Medical Education

*†Psychiatric Research and the Assessment of Change (GAP Report 63, 1966), Formulated by the Committee on Research

*Psychopathological Disorders in Childhood: Theoretical Considerations and a Proposed Classification (GAP Report 62, 1966), Formulated by the Committee on Child Psychiatry

*Laws Governing Hospitalization of the Mentally Ill (GAP Report 61, 1966), Formulated by the Committee on Psychiatry and Law

*Sex and the College Student (GAP Report 60, 1965), Formulated by the Committee on the College Student

*†Psychiatry and the Aged: An Introductory Approach (GAP Report 59, 1965), Formulated by the Committee on Aging

*†Medical Practice and Psychiatry: The Impact of Changing Demands (GAP Report 58, 1964), Formulated by the Committee on Public Education

Psychiatric Aspects of the Prevention of Nuclear War (GAP Report 57, 1964), Formulated by the Committee on Social Issues

*Mental Retardation: A Family Crisis—The Therapeutic Role of the Physician (GAP Report 56, 1963), Formulated by the Committee on Mental Retardation

*Public Relations: A Responsibility of the Mental Hospital Administrator (GAP Report 55, 1963), Formulated by the Committee on Hospitals

*The Preclinical Teaching of Psychiatry (GAP Report 54, 1962), Formulated by the Committee on Medical Education

*Psychiatrists as Teachers in Schools of Social Work (GAP Report 53, 1962), Formulated by the Committee on Psychiatry and Social Work

The College Experience: A Focus for Psychiatric Research (GAP Report 52, 1962), Formulated by the Committee on the College Student

*Toward Therapeutic Care: A Guide for Those Who Work With the Mentally Ill (GAP Report 51, 1961), Formulated by the Committee on Therapeutic Care

*Problems of Estimating Changes in Frequency of Mental Disorders (GAP Report 50, 1961), Formulated by the Committee on Preventive Psychiatry

*Reports in Psychotherapy: Initial Interviews (GAP Report 49, 1961), Formulated by the Committee on Therapy

*Psychiatry and Religion: Some Steps Toward Mutual Understanding and Usefulness (GAP Report 48, 1960), Formulated by the Committee on Psychiatry and Religion

*Preventive Psychiatry in the Armed Forces: With Some Implications for Civilian Use (GAP Report 47, 1960), Formulated by the Committee on Governmental Agencies

*Administration of the Public Psychiatric Hospital** (GAP Report 46, 1960), Formulated by the Committee on Hospitals

*Confidentiality and Privileged Communication in the Practice of Psychiatry** (GAP Report 45, 1960), Formulated by the Committee on Psychiatry and Law

*The Psychiatrist and His Roles in a Mental Health Association** (GAP Report 44, 1960), Formulated by the Committee on Public Education

*Basic Considerations in Mental Retardation: A Preliminary Report** (GAP Report 43, 1959), Formulated by the Committee on Mental Retardation

*Some Observations on Controls in Psychiatric Research** (GAP Report 42, 1959), Formulated by the Committee on Research

*Working Abroad: A Discussion of Psychological Attitudes and Adaptation in New Situations** (GAP Report 41, 1958), Formulated by the Committee on International Relations

*Small Group Teaching in Psychiatry for Medical Students** (GAP Report 40, 1958), Formulated by the Committee on Medical Education

*The Psychiatrist's Interest in Leisure-Time Activities** (GAP Report 39, 1958), Formulated by the Committee on Public Education

The Diagnostic Process in Child Psychiatry (GAP Report 38, 1958), Formulated by the Committee on Child Psychiatry

*Emotional Aspects of School Desegregation** (an abbreviated and less technical version of Report No. 37) (GAP Report 37A, 1960), Formulated by the Committee on Social Issues

*Psychiatric Aspects of School Desegregation** (GAP Report 37, 1957), Formulated by the Committee on Social Issues

*The Person With Epilepsy at Work** (GAP Report 36, 1957), Formulated by the Committee on Psychiatry in Industry

*The Psychiatrist in Mental Health Education: Suggestions on Collaboration With Teachers** (GAP Report 35, 1956), Formulated by the Committee on Public Education

*The Consultant Psychiatrist in a Family Service Agency** (GAP Report 34, 1956), Formulated by the Committee on Psychiatry and Social Work

*Therapeutic Use of the Self (A Concept for Teaching Patient Care)** (GAP Report 33, 1955), Formulated by the Committee on Psychiatric Nursing

*Considerations on Personality Development in College Students** (GAP Report 32, 1955), Formulated by the Committee on the College Student

*Trends and Issues in Psychiatric Residency Programs (GAP Report 31, 1955), Formulated by the Committee on Medical Education

*Report on Homosexuality With Particular Emphasis on This Problem in Governmental Agencies (GAP Report 30, 1955), Formulated by the Committee on Governmental Agencies

*The Psychiatrist in Mental Health Education (GAP Report 29, 1954), Formulated by the Committee on Public Education

*The Use of Psychiatrists in Government in Relation to International Problems (GAP Report 28, 1954), Formulated by the Committee on International Relations

*Integration and Conflict in Family Behavior (Reissued in 1968 as No. 27A) (GAP Report 27, 1954), Formulated by the Committee on Family

*Criminal Responsibility and Psychiatric Expert Testimony (GAP Report 26, 1954), Formulated by the Committee on Psychiatry and Law

*Collaborative Research in Psychopathology (GAP Report 25, 1954), Formulated by the Committee on Psychopathology

*Control and Treatment of Tuberculosis in Mental Hospitals (GAP Report 24, 1954), Formulated by the Committee on Hospitals

*Outline to Be Used as a Guide to the Evaluation of Treatment in a Public Psychiatric Hospital (GAP Report 23, 1953), Formulated by the Committee on Hospitals

*The Psychiatric Nurse in the Mental Hospital (GAP Report 22, 1952), Formulated by the Committee on Psychiatric Nursing—Committee on Hospitals

*The Contribution of Child Psychiatry to Pediatric Training and Practice (GAP Report 21, 1952), Formulated by the Committee on Child Psychiatry

*The Application of Psychiatry to Industry (GAP Report 20, 1951), Formulated by the Committee on Psychiatry in Industry

*Introduction to the Psychiatric Aspects of Civil Defense (GAP Report 19, 1951), Formulated by the Committee on Governmental Agencies

*Promotion of Mental Health in the Primary and Secondary Schools: An Evaluation of Four Projects (GAP Report 18, 1951), Formulated by the Committee on Preventive Psychiatry

*The Role of Psychiatrists in Colleges and Universities (GAP Report 17, 1951), Formulated by the Committee on Academic Education

*Psychiatric Social Work in the Psychiatric Clinic (GAP Report 16, 1950), Formulated by the Committee on Psychiatry and Social Work

*Revised Electro-Shock Therapy Report (GAP Report 15, 1950), Formulated by the Committee on Therapy

*The Problem of the Aged Patient in the Public Psychiatric Hospital
(GAP Report 14, 1950), Formulated by the Committee on Hospitals
*The Social Responsibility of Psychiatry: A Statement of Orientation
(GAP Report 13, 1950), Formulated by the Committee on Social Issues
*Basic Concepts in Child Psychiatry (GAP Report 12, 1950), Formulated
by the Committee on Child Psychiatry
*The Position of Psychiatrists in the Field of International Relations
(GAP Report 11, 1950), Formulated by the Committee on Interna-
tional Relations
*Psychiatrically Deviated Sex Offenders (GAP Report 10, 1950), Formu-
lated by the Committee on Forensic Psychiatry
*The Relation of Clinical Psychology to Psychiatry (GAP Report 9,
1949), Formulated by the Committee on Clinical Psychology
*An Outline for Evaluation of a Community Program in Mental Hy-
giene (GAP Report 8, 1949), Formulated by the Committee on Coop-
eration With Lay Groups
*Statistics Pertinent to Psychiatry in the United States (GAP Report 7,
1949), Formulated by the Committee on Hospitals
*Research on Prefrontal Lobotomy (GAP Report 6, 1948), Formulated by
the Committee on Research
*Public Psychiatric Hospitals (GAP Report 5, 1948), Formulated by the
Committee on Hospitals
*Commitment Procedures (GAP Report 4, 1948), Formulated by the
Committee on Forensic Psychiatry
*Report on Medical Education (GAP Report 3, 1948), Formulated by the
Committee on Medical Education
*The Psychiatric Social Worker in the Psychiatric Hospital (GAP Report
2, 1948), Formulated by the Committee on Psychiatric Social Work
*Shock Therapy (GAP Report 1, 1947), Formulated by the Committee on
Therapy
Index to GAP Publications #1–#80

Symposia Reports

The Right to Die: Decision and Decision Makers (S-12, 1973), Formulated by the Committee on Aging
*Death and Dying: Attitudes of Patient and Doctor (S-11, 1965), Formu-
lated by the Committee on Aging

*Urban America and the Planning of Mental Health Services (S-10, 1964), Formulated by the Committee on Preventive Psychiatry
*Pavlovian Conditioning and American Psychiatry (S-9, 1964), Formulated by the Committee on Research
*Medical Uses of Hypnosis (S-8, 1962), Formulated by the Committee on Medical Education
*Application of Psychiatric Insights to Cross-Cultural Communication (S-7, 1961), Formulated by the Committee on International Relations
*The Psychological and Medical Aspects of the Use of Nuclear Energy (S-6, 1960), Formulated by the Committee on Social Issues
*Some Considerations of Early Attempts in Cooperation Between Religion and Psychiatry (S-5, 1958), Formulated by the Committee on Psychiatry and Religion
*Methods of Forceful Indoctrination: Observations and Interviews (S-4, 1957), Formulated by the Committee on Social Issues
*Factors Used to Increase the Susceptibility of Individuals to Forceful Indoctrination: Observations and Experiments (S-3, 1956), Formulated by the Committee on Social Issues
*Illustrative Strategies for Research in Psychopathology in Mental Health (S-2, 1956), Formulated by the Committee on Psychopathology
*Considerations Regarding the Loyalty Oath as a Manifestation of Current Social Tension and Anxiety (S-1, 1954), Formulated by the Committee on Social Issues

Films

*Discussion Guide to the Film (2, 1970)
*A Nice Kid Like You (1, 1970)

Index

*Page numbers printed in **boldface** type refer to tables or figures.*